THE
Hundred Year
DIET

AMERICA'S VORACIOUS
APPETITE
FOR LOSING WEIGHT

SUSAN YAGER

RODALE

Rodale books may be purchased for business or promotional use or for special sales. For
information, please write to:

Special Markets Department, Rodale Inc., 733 Third Avenue, New York, NY 10017

Printed in the United States of America

Rodale Inc. makes every effort to use acid-free ∞, recycled paper ♻.

Book design by Joanna Williams

Library of Congress Cataloging-in-Publication Data

Yager, Susan.
    The hundred year diet : America's voracious appetite for losing weight / Susan
Yager.
        p.   cm.
    Includes bibliographical references and index.
    ISBN-13: 978-1-60529-011-9   hardcover
    ISBN-10: 1-60529-011-4   hardcover
    1. Weight loss—United States—History.   2. Reducing diets—United States—
History.   3. Weight loss preparations industry—United States—History.   I. Title.
RM222.2.Y24   2010
613.2'5—dc22   2010005873

Distributed to the trade by Macmillan

2   4   6   8   10   9   7   5   3   1   hardcover

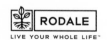

We inspire and enable people to improve their lives and the world around them

For more of our products visit **rodalestore.com** or call 800-848-4735

*For my husband,
dinner and workout partner,
and love of my life, Bob*

CONTENTS

FOREWORD

SIX YEARS AGO MY UNCLE AND HIS GIRLFRIEND (BOTH ON DIETS) AND MY SON AND his wife (who is a vegan) were coming to our house for dinner. Since this was late summer on the east end of Long Island, I had a lot of wonderful, local, animal-free options. I roasted Japanese eggplants for a tomato-eggplant casserole, made a big green salad, sliced some additional heirloom tomatoes, chopped garlic for a simple olive oil and basil pasta, baked some biscotti, and had a lot of fresh peaches, plums, and nectarines ready to grill for dessert. I thought this menu would please the whole crowd. But when my uncle and his girlfriend arrived, they looked at what I was cooking with a combination of panic and horror and sorrowfully announced that there was not a thing they could eat—not a single thing. They needed meat.

They were "on Atkins."

Why didn't they tell my husband or me about this earlier? Because that summer *everyone* was on Atkins, they said, and they'd figured they would just eat the protein. Did we have any cheese?

I had to do something fast and easy, and so decided to put some chickens on the grill, which is not necessarily as fast and easy as it sounds. We are on an island, and our local supermarket had a very small supply of organic, free-range chickens, which was what I wanted. Fortunately, I got to the market in time to purchase the last two birds.

I rubbed them with olive oil, seasoned them, stuffed quartered lemons and lots of fresh herbs in their cavities and pushed garlic under their skins, put them on the grill, opened a bottle or two of wine, and an hour or so later we had a pretty good meal. Two people had chicken plus a loosely packed cup of undressed salad greens, which is the pitifully small amount Atkins allows, and sparkling water. The vegan had everything except the chicken and biscotti, including a few glasses of wine. I've since learned that white wine isn't vegan because eggs whites are generally used in the clarification process, but even if I'd known this then, I probably wouldn't have said anything. The rest of us ate and drank everything in sight.

The next day, a close friend told me he had just begun a diet based on blood type, the theory being that each type—A, B, O, and AB—reacts positively or negatively with certain foods, and if you just learn what they are, you'll get healthy and lose weight. I said this seemed doubtful because there are only four blood types and the majority of the population is either type A or O. He said it had to be better than Atkins.

I started to pay a lot more attention to friends and acquaintances who were on diets. Many had struggled with weight for years, maybe all of their lives. They gained, and then they starved themselves on some new diet, joined a gym, or swallowed supplements they hoped would work like magic. Some had temporary success due to the calorie restriction, exercise, or artificially quickened metabolism; became as hopeful as Liza singing "Maybe This Time"; and then usually ended up gaining back the weight. Their determination and flexibility amazed me—they were so willing to try these dietary distinctions that are in fact all variations on the same principle: taking in fewer calories (or swallowing speed with a fancy name). Some of the ideas were nonsensical. Can anyone really believe that eating by blood type, consuming only grapefruit, or eliminating a life-sustaining nutrient from your diet is the route to long-term health? Why, I wondered, were so many smart people on foolish diets? How did we ever get to the point where two-thirds of the population in the United States need to be on a diet at all? *Do* they need to be? Do some weight-loss schemes that seem absurd, at least to me, really work? Those were the questions swirling around in my brain . . . along with what to have for lunch.

By the way, I've been on a diet ever since I memorized a little blue calorie counter when I was 12 years old.

INTRODUCTION

DINNER IS BEING SERVED. YOUNG WOMEN WITH BEAUTIFUL, CLEAR COMPLEXIONS, bright eyes, and abundant good health are waiting on "invalids" seated at long wooden tables. This scenario has the potential for communal dining at its best—convivial conversation and laughter turning casual acquaintances into friends—but if it weren't for the sounds of eating, the opulent dining hall would be silent. Talk is difficult because everyone is chewing profusely, at least 100 times before swallowing each mouthful, and then meticulously jotting down the portion size and weight for every food choice made. This eating is serious business, and joyless. What must be accomplished is explained clearly: "Cut calories to one-half of normal number until loss of flesh has been secured," and "Fletcherize," which means gnashing all food to a liquid pulp before swallowing it. This part is essential—banners proclaiming FLETCHERIZE! hang at either end of the room.

John D. Rockefeller Jr. might be carefully masticating and calculating at one of these tables, or Thomas Alva Edison, or Henry Ford—powerful men who are usually in complete control of everyone they come in contact with. Here, they are only in control of their own bodies and souls. A few women are dining as well, like the famous dancer Ruth St. Denis and the wife of author Upton Sinclair. There is no need to be concerned about any flirtation; the diners are far too busy worrying about what to choose from the menu. Will it be fruit soup or navy bean, nuttolene fricassee or roast of protose, lettuce salad or potato, graham crackers or Passover bread, sliced bananas or assorted nuts? The year is 1909, and it's dinnertime at the Battle Creek Sanitarium in Michigan, the largest and most luxurious facility of its kind in the world. The richest and most powerful American women—and men—are on a diet.

Bodies and souls are the business of "the San," as its wealthy patrons affectionately call it. Its director, John Harvey Kellogg, MD, is a short, stocky, and charismatic man—surgeon, inventor, vegetarian, and devout Seventh-Day Adventist. He is a philanthropist, but also an astute capitalist who can spot a moneymaking trend when he sees one. He is certain that helping people get rid of a few extra pounds can be a profitable business, and if he can proselytize at the same time, well, that's even better.

GAINED A FEW POUNDS? BANT!

Middle- and upper-class Americans became interested in losing weight in the 1880s, lured by a pamphlet self-published 20 years earlier by an obese Englishman named William Banting that first achieved great popularity in the United Kingdom. Recommended by physicians who thought the tactics it urged were a better choice than taking a little cocaine before meals to curb the appetite (a popular trick), *Letter on Corpulence, Addressed to the Public* was America's first diet book. It was a high-protein, low-calorie, low-fat, modified carbohydrate plan.

Banting, an affluent coffin maker in his sixties, was 5 feet 5 inches tall and weighed 202 pounds when he entered the Soho Square, London, office of aural surgeon Dr. William Harvey. It was a struggle for him to tie his shoes or walk up a flight of stairs, and his hearing was seriously impaired. Banting had already visited numerous physicians but had no luck. Harvey had been researching the effects of obesity on disease and believed that weight reduction would restore hearing and cure rheumatism and gout as well. He instructed his new patient, Mr. Banting, to follow his diet plan carefully.

This plan was so successful that Banting lost 35 pounds in 38 weeks. His hearing was restored, and with his "personal appearance greatly improved" and "all symptoms of indigestion vanished," he felt obligated to share Dr. Harvey's knowledge with the world. At his own expense he wrote, published, and distributed pamphlets describing Harvey's miraculous diet.

This diet required abstinence from "starch and saccharine matter" and included a short list of prohibited foods: bread, butter, milk, sugar, beer, and potatoes. On the Harvey-Banting diet, you eliminated the bread *and* the butter. Banting wrote that these foods had been "the main elements in my subsistence."* His meals were now quite different, consisting of lean meats or fish, biscuits, dry toast, vegetables, fruits, tea without milk or sugar, and copious quantities of "good claret, sherry, or Madeira." He was also allowed a nightcap of one or two glasses of claret or, if preferred, a tumbler of gin. Breakfast consisted of 4 or 5 ounces of lean meat, tea, and 1 ounce of dry toast, which Banting recommended be softened in "a tablespoon of spirit."

This was a new way of living for Banting. He lost weight, of course, but not because of any special diet. He was consuming fewer calories. He continued to follow the diet and write about his progress in subsequent pamphlets. These became so popular that he had to charge a small purchase price to cover his publishing costs, though he donated all of his profits to charity.

As the desire to "reduce" began to sweep the Western world, Banting's book was translated into German. It was well received and became a fashionable alternative to a diet being offered by German physician Wilhelm Ebstein. Banting's plan restricted fatty meats and butter, while Ebstein—a regular 19th-century Robert Atkins—believed that only carbohydrates from sugar and starch turned into fat, while the fat in foods (including bacon) actually made pounds disappear. The Ebstein diet was translated into English and sold to the American market.

Both plans were far from spartan, as calories had not yet been identified and were therefore of no concern. Harvey, Banting, and Ebstein were simply attempting to reduce the consumption of foods that heavier people were thought to eat a lot of. In Harvey's case, they were the foods that his patient, Banting, had previously subsisted on. In other words, these were weight-loss plans based on observation rather than evidence.

Though Ebstein's plan may have been the more appealing one to the average dieter since it allowed butter and other fatty foods, it was

---

*The key to success was the elimination of sugar, milk, and, most important of all, butter, which was by far the dominant cooking fat at that time in both the United Kingdom and America. Take away butter, sugar, and milk, and desserts disappear. Without butter, meats and fish are broiled instead of sautéed or fried, and fresh bread isn't missed nearly as much. Pork and other fatty meats were not allowed, either. It turns out that what Harvey and therefore Banting believed was a diet low in "starch and saccharine matter" was, in fact, a high-protein, *lower*-fat, *lower*-carbohydrate diet. But it is due to Harvey's statement that "starch and saccharine tend to create fat" that Banting's plan is frequently referred to—erroneously—as the first low-carb diet.

Banting who became the star. He had been first on the diet scene; he wasn't foreign; and, unlike Ebstein, who restricted alcohol consumption to three glasses of "light wine" a day, Banting allowed and even encouraged the consumption of most types of alcohol. The word "banting" became the popular term for dieting for the next 50 years.

NO BANTING AT THE SAN

Dr. Kellogg's patients adhered to a much stricter regimen. A Seventh-Day Adventist, he incorporated into it the religion's rigid dietary restrictions—no meat, condiments, leavened bread, alcohol, or caffeine. Like many other intellectuals, social reformers, and religious fundamentalists of the time, Kellogg believed optimal health could only be achieved with a vegetarian and ascetic approach to diet, along with some exercise. For this latter endeavor he used "water cures," vibrating chairs, and roller contraptions of his own design to get the job done. However, he had no evidence that any of it would result in weight loss, which, as a scientist, concerned him.

Soon all of that would change. At the turn of the century, chemists discovered a way to measure the amount of energy, or "calories," in food.

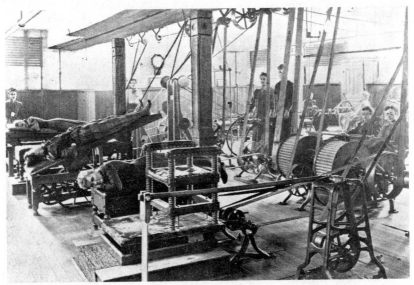

Exercise at the San (Battle Creek Sanitarium Swedish Treatment Room, circa 1900). (Image courtesy of Willard Library, Battle Creek, Michigan)

It became evident that if you ate more "energy" than required to maintain your current weight, you gained pounds, whereas if you ate less, you lost them. This was an amazing and wonderful revelation to Dr. Kellogg. It was so easy—all you needed was self-control.

The San served up a balanced and healthy if painfully boring choice of foods, because Kellogg believed that meat, spicy foods, cheese, coffee, tea, and alcohol resulted in uncontrollable sexual impulses as well as gastrointestinal problems. Breads were "unfermented" because yeast breads, which had to be sensuously kneaded before they tripled in bulk as if impregnated, were far too sexy. "Wine" was also unfermented; in other words, it was grape juice. "Roasts" were nut- and grain-based concoctions resembling what we might today call "meat substitutes." "Coffee" was brewed from cereal grains, not coffee beans. If visiting journalists or other nonpatients requested meats or condiments, they would be accommodated, but they had to sit at the Sinner's Table.

Food and religion, food and science, food and business, food and pretense, food and sin—the legacy of John Harvey Kellogg and other 19th-century social reformers, religious fanatics, and industrialists is still with us when we eat dinner today. Banting and Ebstein are also at the table, their weight-loss schemes transformed and multiplied into methods they could never have imagined.

Today, sitting down to a meal of fresh, wholesome foods simply prepared and enjoying every mouthful doesn't seem possible. Inextricably entangled with commerce, technology, and fear, it has become difficult for many Americans to recognize and appreciate good food. We are confused. We flit from one loopy, illogical diet to the next. We feel guilty; we binge and we purge. And we've become just about the fattest people on Earth.

The purpose of this book is not to explore every weight-loss method devised in the last 100 years, which would become repetitive and probably take at least another century to compile. Instead, this book will concentrate on the most influential people, products, companies, and plans that circumvented what should have been a simple and easy gift in a country where food is mercifully plentiful and varied—and has the capacity to nourish its citizens safely and well.

PART ONE

THE FOUNDING

FATHERS

1

SEX, INDIGESTION, AND WEIGHT LOSS

IN THE MID-1800S, WHEN AMERICA WAS EMERGING AS AN URBAN, INDUSTRIAL, CAPITALIST society and a new science called nutrition was in its infancy, health, sex, morality, and God all became bundled together in unexpected places, including at the dinner table. This rapidly changing world produced a bumper crop of reformers, including abolitionists, temperance seekers, feminists, and religious leaders. Each of these groups held different views on different topics, but one thing they agreed upon, for a period spanning about 60 years, was diet. To be specific: a spare, vegetarian, alcohol- and salt-free diet. That is not to suggest that every agent for change was a vegetarian teetotaler, but the majority at least paid lip service to the idea. Before America became Fast Food Nation, Low-Carb Nation, or even Fat-Free Nation, it was Ascetic Nation, which established a strong foundation for later food fads and gimmicks to build upon.

The equation that a meager and meatless diet resulted in a sound mind and body gained tremendous impetus in 1832, when America experienced its first widespread epidemic: cholera. The popular lecturer, writer, and Presbyterian minister Sylvester Graham, an advocate for temperance and chastity, used the disease to illustrate how a debauchery-filled lifestyle and diet could lead to illness and death, citing as evidence the lascivious ways of cholera-stricken prostitutes in Paris and homosexual young men in India. This made sense to his numerous followers. Cholera, after all, was widespread in urban areas. It had entered the country in New York City via steamship from Europe and was traveling

3

up and down the eastern seaboard. Cholera appeared to be a disease engendered by the Industrial Revolution; it followed commerce and traffic congestion along the new railroad tracks. Unknown at the time (and not to become common knowledge for decades) was the rudimentary fact that cholera was caused by a tiny, comma-shaped bacterium that flourished in and spread via contaminated food and water supplies.

An intense fellow with sunken cheeks, thin lips, and a hawklike beak of a nose, Graham was suspicious of the Industrial Revolution's effects on the food supply—including the increasingly common use of food additives and bleached white flour in mass-produced breads. Graham, a crusader for an old-fashioned and natural way of life, believed that diet and social issues were closely intertwined. If what you ate—or didn't eat—could make you feel better, he reasoned, then certainly your diet could make you (and America) morally better. As correspondent J. M. Bishop stated in a *New York Times* article of the time: "It tends toward a purer spirit in man, ridding the mind of evil thoughts and evil temper, and the body of vicious and ungovernable impulses."

Graham's ultimate mission was to save souls from what he deemed the most serious problem of all: the evil torment of gluttony, which he believed led to sexual excess, violence, and masturbation. Early in his career, Graham wrote: "Treat your stomach like a well governed child; carefully find out what is best for it, as the digestive organ of your body, and then teach it to conform to your regimen."

Graham reasoned that if foods weren't particularly palatable, people would be less likely to eat to excess and misbehave. A Graham diet, therefore, eliminated that beloved staple of the American diet—meat—along with alcohol, coffee, tea, and flavor enhancers such as salt, pepper, and spices. Skeptical of mass-produced, bleached white flour and uncomfortable with the concept of yeast—which, because it fermented, fed on sugar, and multiplied, he (correctly) regarded as a living thing—Graham created an alternative that would become his legacy to culinary history: the unleavened, unsalted, whole-wheat cracker meant to be consumed only after becoming stale. In other words, the graham cracker.

Graham's theory that pure water, bland food, temperance, and chastity could prevent cholera (and other diseases) was partially correct and widely accepted. But there were other frightening problems with our mid-

4

19th-century food supply and eating habits. Lack of refrigeration meant that food spoiled quickly, and the chemical "preservatives" added to prevent (or more likely conceal) spoilage—such as formaldehyde and borax—caused chronic and widespread gastrointestinal pain and, occasionally, death. And then, for the nonreformers, there was overeating. Until the early 20th century, carrying around a few extra pounds was considered a badge of financial success and good health. People didn't even *think* about losing just a little bit of weight. Proper meals often contained as many as 10 courses. A typical breakfast for male private-college students in 1830 consisted of two servings of meat, bread, potatoes, pickles, eggs, toast, hotcakes, biscuits, and butter. And it wasn't only the young and the wealthy who ate with abandon; the middle and working classes had access to a cheap and abundant food supply that placed a heavy emphasis on meat. By 1870, Robert Tomes, writing on the typical American diet, noted: "The national stomach is kept in a constant state of active assault. This overstrains its energy, and produces that malady so common with us which the doctors call atonic dyspepsia." Dyspepsia (a term used to describe a combination of intestinal problems, including stomachache, constipation, and flatulence) and indigestion were major health complaints of the day, problems that were likely intensified for corset-wearing women.

Grahamites who had found relief from their digestive problems by following Graham's vegetarian, whole grain, and essentially sound if painfully boring diet had their testimonials published in *The Graham Journal of Health and Longevity.* One enthusiastic (and typical) Graham follower wrote: "I lived as other folks live, suffering most severely in the stomach. I was always fond of the fattest kinds of meats and richest gravies. In June 1836, I commenced living on the Graham system . . . and sir; from this mode of living I experienced the most happy effects. My health began immediately to improve. I would add that I find fewer occasions for drink than when in the habits of using meats and other excitable foods or condiments." The writer doesn't mention any loss of libido (drinking less alcohol and eating fewer calories probably had the opposite effect than the one Graham intended), but as far as he was concerned, Graham delivered the goods. He no longer suffered from indigestion.

The reverend also had his detractors. When he made a speech at Boston's Marlborough Hotel, the first American "temperance house," police had to intervene when local butchers and bakers, who understandably were not loyal Grahamites, rioted. Journalists nicknamed him the Peristaltic Persuader. When, in 1837, he wrote a series of *Lectures on the Science of Human Life,* the works became the textbooks of a new generation of social reformers, even if some of them, like Mary Gove Nichols and other early feminists, held beliefs antithetical to his own. (It is easy to understand why women's-rights activists were Graham supporters. He was one of the first to hold lecture groups for women only, the main purpose of which was to discuss issues of female anatomy and health. He spoke in favor of brushing the teeth daily and bathing weekly, new and pleasant concepts. His followers could pick and choose: Feminists could throw out the chastity but keep the anatomy lessons, diet, and bathwater.)

The one thing most of Graham's followers (including Susan B. Anthony, Horace Greeley, Amelia Bloomer, Mary Gove Nichols, and Amos Bronson Alcott, educator and father of Louisa May) seemed to agree on was diet. The young, urban, and educated began to follow Graham; soon, university students successfully demanded "Graham board," or vegetarian, meal plans in their dining halls. Graham hotels and boarding houses opened in New York and Boston; shops that sold Graham diet provisions were early versions of today's "health food" stores. Grahamites were youthful, affluent, and, as a result of a diet rich in fruits, vegetables, and whole grains, thin. Today a marketing executive would strive to reach this demographic—the alpha group admired and imitated by others.

Graham died in Northampton, Massachusetts, in 1851, at the age of 57, of "a feeble condition . . . and many deviations from the system he so advocated" according to an obituary, leaving behind a financially secure widow, an 18-year-old son, and a married daughter. His writings and lectures began widespread dietary reforms that still reverberate in demands for pure water and "whole" foods and in the vegetarian and vegan movements.

And so there was much real and perceived good to come from changing the way America ate—and a lot of money to be made.

WHOLE FOODS

James White, an elder in the newly formed Seventh-Day Adventist church, was a direct descendant of Peregrine White, the first child to be born among the Puritan colonists who came to America on the *May-flower*. In 1846 he married Ellen Harmon, an 18-year-old prone to visions and a convert to his church.

Ellen and her identical twin Elizabeth were born near Portland, Maine, in 1827. The girls were 10 years old when a schoolmate threw a rock at Ellen, hitting her on the nose so forcibly that she was knocked unconscious and languished in a critical condition for more than 3 weeks. Her face was badly scarred; she could breathe only through her mouth for the next 2 years; and her ability to concentrate was so diminished that she dropped out of school. Her days were spent resting and performing mundane chores.

Ellen's world changed irrevocably in 1840, when William Miller visited Portland. Miller was the founder of a new Christian sect that predicted the second coming (or "advent") of Christ would occur on the specific date of October 22, 1844. The day she would be carried off to heaven in the arms of Christ couldn't come soon enough for the morose and disfigured young girl who had been raised a Methodist. Ellen converted and became a devout Millerite. When Jesus failed to appear on schedule (the "Great Disappointment" of October 22), Ellen—unlike the majority of her cobelievers—kept the faith.

She met her much older and equally devout husband-to-be, James White, through the Millerite church. The certainty that Christ would reappear on Earth (though perhaps not on a determinable date), along with the return to holding Saturday as the Sabbath, the refusal to bear arms or engage in violence, and the belief in the Old and New Testaments as fact, were the original tenets of their faith.

The Whites began to travel the country in an attempt to unify small groups of followers awaiting their savior. In 1863, they were praying with a small congregation in Ostego, Michigan, when, in mid-prayer, Sister Ellen White fell to the ground in the throes of a vision. Meat, alcohol, tobacco, spices, condiments, coffee, and tea were to be eliminated from the diet, she said, which was to be composed only of fruits, vegetables, and whole grains—the essence of Grahamism. And like Graham, Sister White preached that this vegan, temperate lifestyle would lead to a healthy body and soul and a mind free of lustful thoughts. The Millerite diet was for lust control.

White was an avid reformer of sexual appetites. In the following year, she wrote *An Appeal to Mothers: The Great Cause of the Physical, Mental,*

1

and Moral Ruin of Many of the Children of Our Time. The cause of childhood degradation was summed up in one word—masturbation—a practice she considered to be "an abomination in the sight of God" punishable by death. She describes the world she inhabits as a miserable place. "Everywhere I looked I saw imbecility, dwarfed forms, crippled limbs, misshapen heads, and deformity of every description," she wrote. If only all those poor, self-abusing, overeating souls had a place to go for help.

Two years later, in Battle Creek, Michigan, she and her husband opened the Western Health Reform Institute, which was named after their Adventist magazine, *The Health Reformer.* The institute ran without a full-time medical professional on staff for 10 years, patiently waiting for the man who was being trained and educated for the job.

COFFEE, TEA, OR ABSTINENCE?

That man was John Harvey Kellogg, born in Tyrone, Michigan, in 1852, just a few months after Sylvester Graham's death. His father, John Preston Kellogg, was a former Baptist teacher and avid disciple of both Graham and White who soon moved his family to Battle Creek, where he founded a successful broom-manufacturing business. He and his wife, Mary, became close friends with James and Ellen White, as well as major contributors to their church. When John Harvey was 12 years old, he became a typesetter for *The Health Reformer.* A few years later he began his higher education with an eye toward becoming the protégé of Ellen White and with a goal of serving the cause.

His medical education was sound; he studied at the University of Michigan and was a Bellevue Medical College–trained surgeon, but he graduated in 1874 not to begin practicing medicine, but rather to become editor of *The Health Reformer.* Two years later he was named director of the institute. As a well-credentialed professional, Kellogg brought scientific credibility to the Whites' organization. He was also the first in a long line of physicians to write about nutrition with a passion for, and limited knowledge of, the subject.

Dr. Kellogg was an eccentric. Usually dressed in pure white, he raised the bar on Adventist and Grahamite ideologies in his evening lectures, proclaiming, "coffee cripples the liver," "tea causes insanity," "bouillon is a veritable solution of poisons," and "sex breeds evil diseases."

8

In Dr. Kellogg's world, sexual desire was the primary cause of all of mankind's woes. Like Sylvester Graham and Ellen White, he believed in abstaining from masturbation and sexual activity outside of marriage. He personally practiced abstinence within marriage as well. When he was 28, he married Ella Eaton; they shared a home, had separate bedrooms, and claimed the marriage was never consummated. Over time, they fostered 42 children and adopted many of them.

Eaton was a nurse, educator, and writer with undergraduate and graduate degrees from Alfred University. She was a perfect fit for what was now commonly and affectionately known as "the San,"

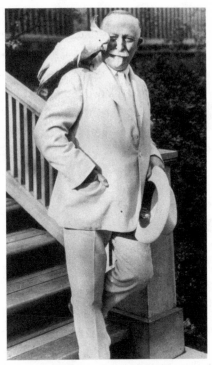

John Harvey Kellogg with cockatoo friend (date unknown). (Image courtesy of Willard Library, Battle Creek, Michigan)

and she wrote numerous articles for *The Health Reformer*. Soon recognizing that the dietary restrictions at the institute made dining unpleasant at best, she began to travel extensively to study cooking techniques. She created alternatives, many of them nut-based, to the food that even John Harvey was beginning to find dull. It was in her test kitchen that peanut butter was created, and also where she and John, in an attempt to create tiny, whole wheat graham crackers, developed a wheat flake cereal that they named Granose. Curiously, these tiny bits of wheat eaten without milk became extremely popular with patients at the San—so popular that they were added to Kellogg's growing line of products from Sanitas, one of the affiliated food companies that manufactured products for sale in grocery stores around the country and shipped products to mail-order customers around the globe. (A few years later, John Harvey's brother Will Keith tinkered with the formula, changing wheat to corn and adding a small bit of sugar. The result was Kellogg's Corn Flakes.)

It should be mentioned that many patients at the San were not actually ill; despite the fact that all visitors were called invalids, truly sick people were discouraged from visiting the beautiful, bucolic, classically proportioned facility on perfectly manicured grounds. Although it was not John and Ellen White's original intent, Kellogg transformed the institute into a place where wealthy people suffering from "wrecked nerves" and "impaired digestion" came for a rest cure or lifestyle change.

NOBODY LOVES A FAT MAN (OR WOMAN)

In 1898, the *Ladies' Home Journal* began a monthly series of "Domestic Lessons," written by Mrs. S. T. Rorer, a home economist and cookbook author. The titles indicate middle-class women's primary concerns of the day: January asked "Do We Eat Too Much Meat?" while February and March focused on the unpleasant and pervasive problems of indigestion. It was not until July that Mrs. Rorer got around to weight. Domestic lesson number seven, "The Best Foods for Stout and Thin Women," suggests that it was unacceptable to be either too thin or too fat. However, the main portion of the "lesson" was devoted to chastising the stout woman. "An excess of flesh is to be looked upon as one of the most objectionable forms of disease, and must be treated as such. Corpulency is naturally the result of excess in partaking of fat-producing foods and a disinclination to exercise." For the woman who was too thin, Mrs. Rorer suggested potatoes, butter, ice cream, and quieting down her "nervous, wiry, constantly on the go" personality. In a very few years, as women's clothing became not only ready-made but also "designed for women of slender figures," the *Ladies' Home Journal* published a piece called "When a Woman Is Stout," which offered helpful hints about how plump women should dress to conceal their shortcomings.

Perceptions of beauty were starting to shift. Those affluent, affable, jolly, "pleasingly plump" people were becoming unhappy, selfish, laughable gluttons. The *Washington Post* ran a heartbreaking story about a father who thought that his 4-foot-tall, 200-pound 12-year-old son had been kidnapped by a local medical school for purposes of weight-loss experimentation. (As it turned out, he wasn't.) In 1906, Roscoe "Fatty"

Arbuckle, a popular actor known for his generous proportions, played a character named Slim who, in an onstage summary of his plight as well as the shifting attitudes in America, says simply and pitifully, "Nobody loves a fat man." In 1910, the *Chicago Daily Tribune* ran an article titled "Are Society Women Literally Killing Themselves to Keep Thin?" stating, "Corpulency is the deadliest enemy of the modern daughter of Eve who desires to be fashionable, and those women who have a tendency to become fat resort to extreme and heroic measures to keep this foe of beauty at bay. They skip rope, roll on the floor, take Turkish baths, and when all else fails it is declared they 'diet' to the point of starvation, ruining health and endangering life for the sake of the svelte figure of youth." Four years later the first reducing salons opened, in Chicago.

WHAT WOULD MAHDAH EAT?

In 1914, the Princeton-educated journalist Vance Thompson wrote *Eat and Grow Thin*, both the first full-length diet book and the first one written by someone who was neither physician nor scientist. Like Banting and the majority of future weight-loss authors, Thompson begins by describing his painful, overweight past: "The worst of being fat is that it makes one ridiculous. . . . The fat man may clown . . . but he is not merry at all; and if one should sink a shaft down to his heart—or drive a tunnel through it—one would discover that it is a sad heart, bleak with melancholy." He saved himself by eating from the "Mahdah Menus." (The unusually named Mahdah is identified only as a female acquaintance whose food plan was based on the dietary charts issued by the USDA. Mahdah may have been a pseudonym for Vance Thompson.) The diet is sophisticated and expensive, recommending plenty of lean meats, shellfish, fruits, and vegetables, but no other carbohydrates. The meals were also complex to prepare. A sample luncheon menu included broiled sweetbreads with stewed celery, quail, endives, and grapefruit; dinner that evening consisted of oyster cocktail, steamed fish, partridges in cabbage, artichokes in vinaigrette, and stewed plums. Breakfast was fresh or stewed fruit, a poached egg once or twice a week, and unsweetened coffee or tea. Calories, not surprisingly, aren't mentioned. What is surprising is that "fletcherizing," the extensive chewing of all foods and a widespread trend of the day, isn't mentioned, either.

DON'T BITE OFF MORE THAN YOU CAN CHEW

In 1895, Horace Fletcher, successful businessman, importer, artist, and epicure, an affluent man of the world, was denied life insurance because he was overweight. His heart might indeed have been bleak with melancholy as he tried various methods to reduce, but all failed. In 1898, he discovered something that worked. He restricted himself to a simple, bland diet—and he masticated. In only 4 months his weight went from 205 to 163, where it remained for the rest of his life. At 5 feet 7 inches and (like John Harvey Kellogg) usually dressed in white, he was now a trim, fit, affluent man of the world with a mission. The Great Masticator, as he quickly became known, believed that ideal health could be attained (and most of mankind's problems solved) by eating less protein and more carbohydrates and fats, but only when very hungry; allowing no depressing thoughts while at the dinner table; chewing multiple times; and not swallowing until the food was liquefied.

In 1902, Russell Chittenden, a well-respected Yale physiologist and early pioneer in nutrition, invited Fletcher to his university to study the amount of food necessary for men to achieve maximum efficiency. Fletcher, who by this time had created hundreds of cards listing the appropriate number of steady and rapid—100 per minute—chews necessary for various foods to be properly pulverized, helped to finance the experiments. The US government donated 13 soldiers, who were, understandably, hostile about having a diet restrictive of both calories and animal protein. However, after 6 months of eating a diet consisting of fewer than 3,000 calories per day and very little meat, they were reported to have flourished, showing a loss of fat and what Chittenden called a "phenomenal gain in muscular power." Then Irving Fisher, PhD, a Yale professor and political economist, experienced such success on a low-protein, meatless, masticating diet that he began some experiments of his own. Believing that enormous gains could be made in human efficiency and the American economy if animal proteins were eliminated or reduced, Fisher began to study the effects of diet on energy. Nine students were permitted to eat whatever they desired as long as they followed Fletcher's precepts. After 6 months, they adjusted themselves to the Chittenden standard, which allowed 60 grams of protein daily for the average male, and they thrived. Fisher summarized: "Our conclusion in brief is that Mr. Fletcher's claims, so far as they relate to endurance, are justified." (He never mentions that if you have to chew endlessly, it might be a lot more pleasant to eat soft food, resulting in less meat and calories consumed.) Fisher's next experiment was a kind of battle of the Titans that pitted athletic flesh-eaters from Yale against vegetarian doctors and nurses from Kellogg's sanitarium. They competed in contests of deep knee bending and holding their arms straight out. The masticating vegetarians won every battle.

Just as millions of dieting Americans in the early 21st century believed the Atkins diet to be a magical way to shed pounds, millions of Americans in the early 20th century believed the way to lose weight and achieve optimal health was to fletcherize. And like the Atkins diet, this fad had staying power. In 1898, the *Ladies' Home Journal* instructed readers that food should be "well masticated." Ten years later, the same magazine stated, "Fletcherism has become a fact. The most famous men of science teach it and endorse its principles." The author Henry James; his philosopher brother, William; and John D. Rockefeller did it. So did Thomas Edison and Henry Ford. Masticating had no social boundaries. Sing-Sing prison inmates, schoolchildren, the highest of high society, and the middle-most of the middle class all chewed and chewed.

The "scientific evidence" (drawn from less than 100 subjects) proving the benefits of multiple chews did not convince everyone. In 1910, the *Washington Post* published a list of "39 False Food Fads." Number 23 says that it is a fallacy that "prolonged mastication should be made a cult." (Number 8 warns of the danger of a carbohydrate-free diet.) And in 1912, Dr. Charles Barker, who wrote a book about happiness, stated: "This chewing your food for 60 and 90 times makes you disgusted with your meals. I do not believe in fletcherizing. It makes you sick of everything you eat." The voice of reason, however, has never been heeded when it comes to mealtime in America. The trend continued to grow. Fletcher was reported as saying that if everyone just fletcherized, there would be "no slums, no degeneracy, no criminals, no policemen, no criminal courts. . . . In a single generation the whole social problem would be solved." Like Graham and

13

Kellogg, Fletcher ultimately became a social reformer, believing that diet determined health, morality, and the future of America.

DR. WILEY'S POISON SQUAD

There was another, darker side to the American diet: What you eat could literally kill you. Until the late 1800s, there were no government agencies to regulate food safety on any level. In 1906, Upton Sinclair published *The Jungle,* a novel that exposed the wretchedly inhumane and unsanitary conditions in Chicago's slaughterhouses. There were other types of food poisoning to be concerned about as well. Prior to refrigeration, putrefaction of many foods was rampant. Suppliers, attempting to prevent or cover up costly decay, dumped a variety of chemicals into the food supply. Harvey Washington Wiley, MD, a chemist who headed up the USDA Bureau of Chemistry (now the FDA) and one of the first people to work on determining the nutrient composition of foods, was concerned that these substances were harmful. In 1902, he began a series of human experiments to prove he was right.

Wiley, born in Kent, Indiana, in 1844, was the son of a struggling farmer and strict Calvinist who believed "religion was the sole end aim of life." In his 1930 autobiography, he describes even Christmas as a "somewhat drab affair in our home, no exchange of presents, no stockings hanging in front of the fire, no turkey dinner." His strongly principled father, whom he adored, was, according to Wiley, the first abolitionist in Jefferson County, and the first conductor on the area's "underground railroad." At a time when votes were cast orally and a man who spoke out against slavery in that part of Indiana risked personal injury and even his life, Wiley's father was the only man in the county to vote for abolitionist Martin Van Buren when he ran for reelection in 1840.

Those early lessons in morality, deprivation, and courage were the underpinnings of Wiley's life. It took a brave man certain of his convictions to begin this unique series of experiments: His Chemical Boarding House, also known as the Borax Café, was where 12 young male chemists, thrilled by their proximity to the famous and well-respected Dr. Wiley, were fed food laced with borax and formaldehyde in gradually increasing

14

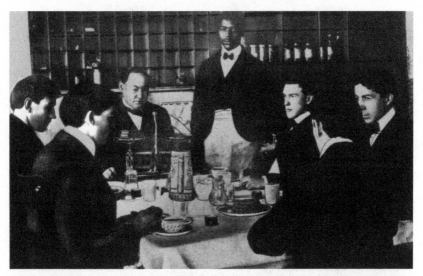

Dr. Harvey W. Wiley and volunteers, officially designated the "Hygienic Table," circa 1905. Dr. Wiley is seated at the center of the table. The man standing at his left is likely William Carter, the first African American chemist at the FDA and at the time "cook" for the Poison Cafe. (Image courtesy of the National Library of Medicine, Bethesda, Maryland)

dosages. Wiley's research objective was to determine the maximum amount of these commonly used additives that could be ingested before toxicity kicked in. Wiley's "Poison Squad" ate poison for years, with new subjects rotating in every 12 months.

By 1907, the Borax Café had attracted the attention of Congress, and Wiley appeared before the House Committee on Expenditures in the Agricultural Department to defend his experimental budgets. Wiley believed that a 150-pound male could eat "one and one half pounds of dry matter on a daily basis if you take the water out of your food and count just the dry matter." He goes on to state what was becoming obvious: "If a man eats less he will lose in weight and if he eats more he will gain in weight." On this basis, the 150-pound male was to ingest exactly $4\frac{1}{2}$ pounds of liquids and solids daily to maintain his exact weight, which was necessary if Wiley was to accurately measure the effects of the preservatives.

These methods may be suspect by today's standards, but Wiley's research disclosed the dangers of untested food additives at a time when there were no government regulations for purity. In 1906, the first Food and Drugs Act was passed, banning interstate shipment of potentially harmful foods, and Wiley was put in charge of enforcement. He eventually became frustrated

15

with the bureaucracy of government work and resigned in 1912. He spent the rest of his life as an activist attacking government food policy and, as head of the Good Housekeeping Research Institute, advocating for pure foods and drugs. He died in 1930, soon after publishing his autobiography.

A lot of Wiley's findings about commonly used preservatives proved alarming; for example, sulfur diminished the blood's ability to carry oxygen throughout the body, while borax damaged the kidneys. The implication was that all foods with chemical additives were harmful—something that Sylvester Graham had suggested decades earlier. Of course the controversy continues, justifiably, until the present day.

A loaf of bread was no longer a loaf of bread. The foundation for food fads and fears was laid by Sylvester Graham and built upon by Banting, Kellogg, Fletcher, and Wiley. Americans were getting accustomed to being told what to eat, what not to eat, and how to eat, even if the information changed on a regular basis.

CALORIES COUNT

An irrevocable change occurred in 1894 when the USDA published its Farmers' Bulletin No. 23, entitled *Foods: Nutritive Value and Cost,* which introduced dietary and nutritional recommendations that would have a major impact on food choice in America for more than a century to come. Compiled by Wilbur Olin Atwater, PhD, a chemistry professor at Wesleyan University and the USDA's first director of research activities, the pamphlet contained composition tables that listed the protein, fat, and "carbohydrate matter" of common foods. Atwater also determined that a gram of protein or carbohydrate had approximately 4 units of energy and a gram of fat had about 9, so simple multiplication provided an energy, or "calorie" (from *calor,* the Latin word for heat), value specific to different foods. Atwater recommended that an American male laborer consume about 3,500 calories per day, 52 percent of it carbohydrates, 33 percent fat, and 15 percent protein. Although this may seem high (the amount of energy expended daily by the average male today is less), the macronutrient breakdown is remarkably similar to the current USDA guidelines of 55 percent carbohydrates, 30 percent fat, and 15 percent protein. In an earlier position statement, Atwater had noted that Americans consumed too much sugar and fat-laden meats and didn't get enough exercise.

FOOD IS SCIENCE, AND SCIENCE IS FOOD

The 1896 first edition of Fannie Merritt Farmer's *Boston Cooking-School Cook Book* began like a textbook, with a breakdown of the 13 elements, by percentage, that were thought to make up the human body. The preface clearly states the newly elevated role of science in determining diet: "During the last decade much time has been given by scientists to the study of foods and their dietetic value, and it is a subject which rightfully should demand much consideration from all. I certainly feel that the time is not far distant when knowledge of the principles of diet will be an essential part of one's education. Then mankind will eat to live." Or, as writer Carl Malmberg would put it 35 years later: A man was no longer just a man; he was a "steam engine in breeches."

The Atwater nutrient composition and calorie charts were what had the greatest immediate impact on the American diet. For the first time, food was quantifiable. John Harvey Kellogg incorporated calories into his 1909 *Battle Creek Sanitarium Diet List,* where he joyfully states: "Dietetics has at long last come to be a science. The properties and values of foods have been studied by the same methods which have determined the qualities and values of soils and ores." And so, for Kellogg and his affluent clients and for Fannie Merritt Farmer and her middle-class housewives, food could at long last be stripped of all mystery, romance, and art, valued only as the sum of scientifically measured parts.

Eight years later, a formerly obese physician named Lulu Hunt Peters would write a book called *Diet and Health, with Key to the Calories.* "Is it a disgrace to be fat?" Peters would ask—and answer: "Not now, for we have not had much popular instruction along the line of dietetics. But it will be a disgrace before long."

She was right. Soon, counting calories would become an American way of life.

2

AMERICA, WHAT'S YOUR WEIGHT?

SHORTLY AFTER THE "DISCOVERY" OF THE CALORIE IN 1894, THE US GOVERNMENT began to instruct citizens on how to wisely spend their personal fuel dollars. School lunch programs were devised to feed children half of their daily caloric needs for three cents. Ten cents' worth of peanuts could feed a male laborer for a day, but he could eat for two with a dime's worth of beans. People were urged to beat the high cost of living by learning how many calories were in foods considered to be of comparative nutritive value, like bacon, turkey, cod, steak, and nuts, and shopping to get the most calorie bang for their buck. The government studied various workers' families' diets, carefully measuring who ate what and compiling this information into composition charts that reflected the nutrients and calories consumed daily. The results were printed in little booklets that were distributed to the public. The overwhelming message was to eat for good health, not for good taste, and as economically as possible: Food is fuel. Many women who aspired to careers in science found one in the new field of scientific nutrition. Some of these home economists, as they were called, had studied with disciples of Wilbur Olin Atwater. They dedicated much of their time to researching and analyzing the diets of immigrant families, with the goal of assimilation via nutrition. Immigrants were encouraged to eat foods that were culturally acceptable, inexpensive, and nutritious. As well intentioned as this idea may have been, it was also terribly misguided. If an Italian family could find imported olive oil, pasta, and good-quality cheese, that became dinner—to many, taste was more important than price. Most Europeans were (and still are) willing to spend a larger percentage of their incomes on food than the number-crunching food reformers anticipated.

Still, long before the fast food revolution of the 1950s, the American diet was beginning to homogenize. If farmhands, factory workers, house-wives, and students were machines that needed fuel, why not spend the least amount of money possible to produce the most energy? It was all spreadsheet analysis, with menus created by the accounting department. Weight didn't enter into this equation for any but the very wealthy; most others thought of calories as highly productive nuggets of energy, if they thought about them at all. But soon a syndicated columnist and physician named Lulu Hunt Peters would change that.

EVEN AS I HAVE SAVED MYSELF, SO WILL I SAVE YOU

Lulu Hunt was born in Milford, Maine, in 1873. As a child, she was an overweight outsider, interested in things other late-Victorian-era girls found repugnant. While her classmates were learning to embroider a tablecloth or frost a cake, Lulu would splash around in brooks, catching frogs she would later dissect. When questioned about her conduct, she replied, "I want to see what they look like inside. And I want to find out what makes 'em move."

This is the childhood behavior of either a sociopath or a scientist, depending upon brain chemistry and background, and Lulu happily became the latter. She graduated from college with honors and earned a medical degree from the University of California in 1909, the year John Harvey Kellogg began counting calories at the San. Her talent for sim-plifying and communicating complex ideas along with her passion for nutrition catapulted Lulu to the highest ranks. She became one of the best-known physicians in America, lecturing on dietetics and the latest methods of weight control with clarity, honesty, and humor.

Hunt married Louis H. Peters shortly after she graduated from medi-cal school, walking down the aisle at 5 feet 7 inches and 165 pounds. Always on the heavy side, her weight in the next few years would balloon to 230

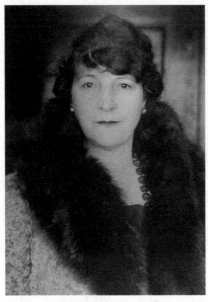

Dr. Lulu Hunt Peters visits Boston, March 28, 1922. It is a crime to be fat—a crime against love, health, efficiency, and society, Peters states on the trip. (Image courtesy of Corbis)

pounds. She was fat and miserable. Later, she wrote about how she resisted losing weight because her husband kept telling her he liked her just the way she was. "I almost hate my husband when I think how long he kept me under that delusion. Now, of course, I know all about his jealous disposition, and how he did not want me to be attractive." Whether or not this is true, Peters was clear about what she wanted to weigh—a reasonable 150 pounds. She determined this by a simple rule: "Multiply number of inches over 5 feet in height by $5\frac{1}{2}$ and add 110. For example, if you are 5 feet 7 inches tall without shoes, your ideal weight is 148.5 pounds."*

This formula was the basis for her 1918 best-selling diet book, *Diet and Health, with Key to the Calories.* Finally, someone was explaining exactly how much you *should* weigh, and how to achieve it. Of course, it wasn't going to be easy. You began with a 3-day liquid fast of 500 to 600 calories a day. There was a penance to be paid, determination and willpower to be tested.

Now fat individuals have always been considered a joke, but you are a joke no longer. Instead of being looked upon with friendly tolerance and amusement, you are now viewed with distrust, suspicion, and even aversion! How dare you hoard fat when our

---

* Although Peters didn't mention the source for this formula, it was based on Belgian mathematician and statistician Adolphe Quetelet's 1835 index correlating height and weight to "average" body size. Quetelet's index is now referred to as the body mass index (BMI), and since the 1970s it has controversially been used to determine underweight, overweight, obesity, and morbid obesity, replacing life insurance charts.

THE FOUNDING FATHERS

nation needs it? You don't dare to any longer. You never wanted to be fat anyway, but you did not know how to reduce. . . .

But cheer up. I will save you; yea, even as I have saved myself and many, many others, so will I save you.

DON'T HELP THE HUN AT MEALTIME

Feeding troops adequately in wartime had always been of concern, but never before had there been such sophisticated knowledge about food as energy—as *calories*. It was now possible to calculate adequate human fuel per cubic inch, the more economically to transport food overseas at first to our allies and then to our troops. Now that it was common knowledge that some foods contained more calories than others, it became sinful to consume too much sugar or fat and to have the waistline to show for it.

Herbert Hoover was appointed federal food administrator in 1916. His administrative and engineering credentials as well as his impressive humanitarian efforts distributing food to the Allies made him a good choice, especially now that it was evident America would soon be sending troops over there, which began in April 1917. His job was to keep the US Armed Forces and Allies well fed, and he repeatedly stated that *victory depended upon food*. "Do not help the Hun at mealtime" was a popular slogan. There could be no eating to excess or wasting of food if we were to suppress the enemy. The British and the French had food rationing plans in place as well (although for the French they were voluntary), but Hoover felt America didn't need any such thing. He demanded that everyone in the country join together, adding, "If democracy is worth anything we can do these things by cooperation. If it cannot be done, it is better that we accept German domination and confess the failure of our political ideals." In the summer of 1918, he took one of his many trips abroad to see how our allies and troops were faring. "All fed!" he reported, congratulating American farmers for their good work and American citizens for their willpower.

An ample supply of "fuel" for our soldiers meant we would win the war, and ubiquitous posters told what must be done:

21

Eat less and let us be thankful that we have enough to share with those who fight for freedom.

Eat more corn, oats and rye products, fish and poultry, fruits, vegetables and potatoes, baked, boiled and broiled foods. Eat less wheat, meat, sugar and fats to save for the army and our allies.

Peters recommended joining together to form "Watch Your Weight Anti-Kaiser" groups, the early, patriotic precursor to Weight Watchers.

This way of eating was a dream come true for the new home economists. Just as the 19th-century food reformers' soul-saving diets would almost guarantee better health and weight loss as unintended consequences, the same resulted from the World War I diet. People were urged to eat less of the foods that packed the most calories because those were the foods that sent the most energy overseas in the smallest amount of space. Fewer calories were consumed on all of those "Meatless Mondays" and "Wheatless Wednesdays" back home.

In just a few years, an overweight person went from being socially acceptable (William Howard Taft, president of the United States from 1909 to 1913, weighed 300 pounds) to being an outcast who took up too much space and used up too many valuable resources. Lulu Hunt Peters's crusade to make America count every calorie coincided with Herbert Hoover's enormous job of keeping the troops well fed. She asked, and received, permission to dedicate her book to him.

Peters's writing style, a combination of humor, tough love, and personal salvation, gave readers an authoritative solution to this widespread new "problem" of obesity. She became America's first successful weight-loss guru.

In 1922, Peters became a columnist for the *Los Angeles Times*, writing a daily piece called "Diet and Health," and soon became one of the best-known syndicated journalists in the country. Her introductory column warned that though the war might be over, a new battle was just beginning: "[Most disease] can be prevented in a large measure by a campaign against one thing—and that one thing is obesity, or to use the short and ugly term, fat! Hurrah. You're with me! I knew it. We're off! What's your weight?"

Peters was the most famous physician to write about weight. But she wasn't the first.

HEALTH IS WEALTH

William Augustus Evans, MD, was born in Marion, Alabama, in 1865 and appointed to the newly created position of public health commissioner for Chicago in 1907. He was a popular civic leader, known as a "confirmed bachelor" until he surprised the town by secretly marrying Ida May Wildberger of Memphis, Tennessee, in the same year. An 1885 graduate of Tulane Medical School, he completed his postgraduate training at the Pasteur Institute in Paris, earned a doctorate in public health, and became a professor of hygiene at Northwestern University in Chicago. A man of varied interests, Evans published a biography of Mary Todd Lincoln, prospected for gold in New Mexico, and traveled extensively in Africa and Asia. Preventive medicine, however, was his passion. His syndicated column, "How to Keep Well," containing the catchphrase "Health Is Wealth," began in the *Chicago Daily Tribune* in 1911, and was notable in that it was the first of its kind to be labeled "disinterested," meaning that Evans would not endorse products or take money from sponsors or advertisers. Over the 23 years that he wrote his popular daily column, he answered more than 1 million questions from readers—albeit often with few words. When a 5-foot-5-inch-tall, 40-year-old motorman inquired how he might lose 30 pounds, Evans responded: "Eat less."

Keeping well—that is, preventing illness today rather than curing it tomorrow—was a revolutionary concept, and Evans was considered to be one of the world's greatest authorities on what is now known as preventive medicine. The *Daily Tribune* advised readers that nothing the paper published would ever be more important than Evans's advice. His columns, printed on the *Daily Tribune*'s editorial page, read today like a history of illness and medicine in the early decades of the 20th century, mixed with the homespun advice of a country doctor. He wrote about the mainly forgotten horrors of diphtheria, typhoid fever, scarlet fever, yellow fever, plague, leprosy, gonorrhea, and syphilis and about diseases that are still with us, like malaria, influenza, and tuberculosis. He wrote about

23

the best way to clean the house. "Anti-vaccinationists" were urged to accept smallpox vaccinations for the sake of all people. Iceboxes didn't come with thermometers, he warned, please put one inside immediately! And from the start, Evans wrote about weight. "Many worry because they are fat, others because they are slim and spare of body. Today we shall take up the bigger proposition . . . obesity is a serious hindrance to the enjoyment and comfort of life." The Evans cure for obesity was simple: "Stop feeding the trouble." Gaining was easy, too—eat more and stop being so fidgety and nervous. In 1912, he printed some unwieldy calorie and protein charts based on Atwater's work for the US Department of Agriculture. Five ounces of meat equaled 400 calories and 60 grams of protein; 180 grains of sugar equaled 50 calories and no protein. Evans recommended two scales for the person who wanted to gain or lose weight—"one to weigh the subject on; one on which to weigh his food"—a popular tactic endorsed by many diet plans today.

On Christmas Eve of 1913, Evans gave his readers the present of a new and improved chart based on a new Atwater booklet. Common foods were finally listed in easy-to-understand portions. A medium apple was 60 calories, a medium banana 50, and a large oyster 10. A lump of sugar was 40 calories, no need to count the granules. Evans even approximated how many calories each family member needed on a daily basis: Father and mother each required 2,500, their 9-year-old boy 1,250, their 6-year-old daughter 1,000, and their 1-month-old baby 500, with no differentiation for sex, height, or occupation. In April of 1915, he printed up-to-date charts from the New York Life Insurance Company's aggregate statistics on policyholders. Life insurance executives had a strong interest in a client's weight since a few studies were already correlating lower weight with longevity. A 20-year-old, 5-foot-4-inch female was considered normal at 123 pounds and obese if more than 148 pounds; at age 55, however, she was normal at 145 pounds and not considered obese unless she weighed 175 pounds or more. A 6-foot-tall man was normal if he was 30 years old and 172 pounds, but obese if he weighed more than 216. At age 55, however, he could weigh 183 pounds and be normal and would have to weigh more than 227 pounds to be labeled obese. The subjects used in drawing up the original charts were customers who wanted insurance and were affluent enough to be able to afford it, a self-selecting group of predominantly white, middle-class men from the eastern seaboard. It is probable that for New York Life's original purpose, "average" wasn't thin enough; below "average" was much preferred.

In 1931, Evans retracted the idea that weight should increase with age. Instead, he believed, a person should maintain the same weight throughout life, a point that is still under debate. Difficult-to-achieve and perhaps unrealistic standards were beginning to be established.

During the 1920s, Evans's gentle attitude toward the obese began to change, and by 1925 the congenial doctor had become cruel. This reflects a shift in the cultural attitude that began around the time America entered World War I and became increasingly prejudicial by the middle of the following decade. "Of each 100 fat jokes," Evans wrote on March 9, 1925, "at least 50 have not the self-control required to reduce. They are just fat jellyfish, calling themselves members of the superior human race." He went on to list the terrible dangers of obesity, which he said included pneumonia, diabetes, kidney disease, difficulty surviving anesthesia, shortness of breath, and premature death. Perhaps the worst danger of all was loneliness, which obese people were subject to, he concluded, because "nobody loves 'em."

In the mid-1920s, Evans, like Peters, believed that most Americans weighed too much.

HEALTH TALKS

Other experts had similar points of view. In 1925, William Brady, MD, the "Health Talks" columnist for the *Atlanta Constitution,* answered questions about weight in the brutal style reminiscent of certain radio talk show hosts today. When someone inquired whether a tendency toward overweight might be inherited, he sarcastically replied:

A good appetite. There you are, fat folks. That's the secret of maintaining the family tradition. It is so very easy to overeat, with all the tempting delicacies of the table and the concentrated calories in the confections served at the soda fountain where the

*fat girls seem to gravitate so much. When you consider how sim-
ple it is to slide 500 calories down the esophagus in the shape of a
chocolate marshmallow nut sundae, and how painfully labori-
ous it is to burn the 500 calories walking several miles or taking
other active exercise, is it any wonder that so many fat people like
to blame it on grandma?*

If you were fat, it was your own damn fault. Excess weight was, in the
words of the beloved Lulu Hunt Peters, "a disgrace."

BUT *WERE* AMERICANS FAT?

Despite the widely accepted new theory that the thinner you were, the longer you would live, people weren't much heavier than they had been in previous decades. Indeed, a lot of Americans still wanted to *gain* weight. Peters
addressed this concern in one of her "Diet and Health" columns, incredulously writing, "How anyone could want to be anything but thin was beyond
my comprehension." However, she did allocate pages in her book and many
lines of copy in her columns to trying to help "yon Cassiuses" attain "normal" weight. "You are going to be my animal, and I am going to be your
farmer," she began one column. "I shall fatten you just as any other farmer
would fatten any other animal."

However, although people were becoming far less tolerant of extra
weight on themselves and others, there are numerous indications that
there wasn't actually all that much extra weight to go around. The 1883
class of men entering Yale averaged about 5 feet 8 inches and weighed
138 pounds; in 1923 they averaged 5 feet 9 inches and weighed 141½
pounds. At 1 inch taller and only 3½ pounds heavier, they were in better shape than the men of 4 decades prior. Young women in the Midwest averaged 5 feet 3 inches and 114 pounds in 1893 and 5 feet 4
inches and 121 pounds in 1933. Using Peters's formula, they were
underweight, and they would be on the low side of normal using the
modern BMI formula.*

---

* You can easily determine your BMI at www.nhlbisupport.com/bmi/bminojs.htm.

THE FOUNDING FATHERS

Americans just didn't weigh all that much in this period before sub-urbs, televisions, computers, minivans, and supersizing. Those who moved from rural lives to apartments in cities probably gained a bit unless they ate fewer calories, but no one wanted to be *too* thin any-way, in a world still dealing with diseases like diphtheria and tuberculosis that caused emaciation. Only a very few years earlier, being "pleasingly plump" had been a positive thing. In 1928, Americans were eating 5 percent *fewer* calories per capita than they had in 1890 and were consuming more green vegetables and citrus fruits and less potatoes and beef. People were taller, better nourished, and healthier than ever before, but when they looked in their mirrors, they saw distorted, fun-house reflections. Our cultural perception of weight was profoundly shifting.

THE NAKED TRUTH ABOUT YOUR WEIGHT

Whether they felt too thin, too fat, or just right, in the 1920s most people knew how much they weighed. Fifty percent of households had indoor plumbing, and many of those bathrooms had scales, allowing a person to undress and weigh him- or herself morning, noon, and night. "To be over or underweight is often detrimental to health! Science has determined the correct weight for everyone, according to height and age and sex," advertised the Detecto Scale Company. "A few pounds underweight and the delectable curves give place to ugly angles. A few pounds over-weight and the graceful contour of youth has become heavy and unpleas-ant," was how the Continental Scale Company brochure put it. Unless you checked a couple of times a day and knew how much you weighed as well as you knew your own name, how could you ever take *control* of your body? You could "safeguard your health" for $12.95 or less, or 50 cents a week, no money down.

Not everyone could afford a scale, of course, especially the half of the population that was without a bathroom containing a flush toilet. But if you couldn't weigh yourself privately, in the nude, at least once a day, you could at least pay a penny to get weighed in public (fully clothed). The life insurance companies' ideal-weight charts took into account the added weight of clothing and shoes. It seems as though just about everyone used penny scales, whether they owned bathroom scales or not. A woman might weigh herself at home in the morning, and then again later in the day at a department store, away from her insensitive, inquiring spouse. In 1927, the *New York Times* said that 500 million persons had stepped onto the platforms of some 40,000 penny scales in the prior year, dropping 500 million pennies into the slots. By 1928, the *Los Angeles Times* reported that 800 million pennies were being spent to "see how the calories are behaving." The wife of the distributor of Roberts Weight-O-Health weighing machines put down a deposit on a new Nash automobile by dropping off sacks stuffed with 30,000 pennies.

Not gaining, not losing, but just *checking* weight had turned into a lucrative business. To maintain privacy, scales no longer had big, round, clocklike faces that could be seen from a distance; instead, your weight (and, as a bonus, your fortune) was printed on a paper ticket. No one had to know the truth but you. And the truth was alarming if you didn't measure up to the "ideal" weight charts that were attached to most scales.

If you were too thin, you could drink the "bodybuilder" called Todd's Tonic, made of the finest California wine and guaranteed to put pounds on you (and give you an elusive buzz during Prohibition). And if you needed to lose a few pounds? Luckily, there were a number of new options available that didn't require you to diet *or* exercise.

BANTING WITH BASY

Quick "cures" with names like Allan's Anti-Fat and Get Slim had been around for decades, but by the 1920s a much wider range of products was becoming available—and people were buying all of them. Although the truth was that there may not have been enough overweight people in America to sustain the weight-loss industry, the perceived need to get thin made that of little consequence. In 1906, Dr. Walter's Famous Medicated Reducing Rubber Garments were advertised in *Vogue*; the company was still running ads in the magazine's 1923 30-year-anniversary issue, with line drawings showing men and women wearing rubber neck and chin reducers, which look as bizarre as they sound, as well as rubber brassieres and anklets. The best-selling item of this group, however, was the rubber girdle—the *New York Times* suggested that it was so comfortable that the "stout woman" wasn't the only one wearing one, most women were. By 1923, Dr. Walter had been joined by Dr. Lawton, who sold a "guaranteed way to rub away fat with a vacuum-suction massage"; Francis Jordan, who sold a kneader to make "the fat roll off"; and "specially formulated" Basy bread that cost a very expensive $1 per loaf but allowed you to "reduce naturally" by eating three slices of the stuff a day and following the Basy Bread Diet, which allowed no potatoes, oils, fats, or sugars.

In an editorial, *Vogue* commented on all of these new weight-loss advertisements and on how times had changed: "Thirty years ago, no one ever talked of reducing; no woman knew what calories were. . . . This is our ideal today. Gone are the busts, the hips, the curves of yesteryear. Woman's figure is the exclamation point of the world!"

THAT COMFORTABLE STATE BETWEEN TWO EXTREMES

"Thin" is a culturally relative term, and at that time, many physicians still recommended that having a little extra flesh in reserve was a good thing in case one developed an infection (many of which were still deadly before the discovery of antibiotics). A former American Medical Association president, Woods Hutchinson, MD, wrote that he found "This present onslaught upon one of the most peaceful, useful, and law-abiding of our tissues"—fat, that is—"puzzling." While some middle- and upper-middle-class folks emulated the wealthy and dieted, many of those who were less well off ignored the whole trend. Others, particularly young college girls who believed that being too thin could pose a hazard to their reproductive health, had all the more reason to eat a second or third serving, even while some of their sorority sisters were on diets. This was the conundrum for the women of Smith College in Northampton, Massachusetts. Beginning in 1917, the school physician gave each new student a detailed Atwater-style composition and calorie chart for various popular foods like ice cream, corn muffins, and lamb stew and an "ideal" height and weight chart. In 1924, three students coauthored a letter to the editor of the *Smith College Weekly* questioning all of the "strenuous dieting" that was going on and stating that they feared "Smith College will become notorious . . . for the haggard faces and the dull, listless eyes of her students."

The tools were readily available to help you reconstruct your body—if you wanted to. It was a nation divided as to whether or not that was necessary, although *Good Housekeeping* in 1924 might have come to a reasonable compromise when it told readers that the ideal was neither thin nor fat, but "that comfortable state between the two extremes."

IF YOU WANT TO LOSE WEIGHT, CHICAGO IS YOUR KIND OF TOWN

However, there was a small percentage of the population that was a long way past that comfortable state, and the media, under the guise of self-help, was ready and willing to profit from its pain. In the early decades of the 20th century, newspapers sometimes created their own news in order to have a big story to follow closely on a daily basis. These serials became a combination of reality shows and soap operas. For example, in 1908 the *New York Times* sponsored and sent correspondents to follow an automobile race that began in Times Square and ended in Paris by way of the frozen Bering Strait. Along the way, the competitors became household names.

In 1920, the New York Daily News–Chicago Tribune Syndicate began a similar type of contest—one that involved different personalities and a large chunk of time. An overweight group of 25 women, led by Chicago health commissioner John Dill Robertson, MD, would compete to see who could lose the most weight. On April 22, the *Chicago Daily Tribune* ran this invitation—not an advertisement, mind you—to audition: "FAT FOLKS! See Dr. Robertson and Grow Thin! He will trim you down. For three weeks, overweight Chicago women will compete."

Many rushed to join the competition. A reporter for the *New York Tribune* who was covering the event indelicately observed, "It looked like a convention of circus heavyweights. The elevator men of the City Hall threw up their hands in horror." The next day, the *Chicago Daily Tribune* ran a picture of Robertson lecturing his 25 overweight and eager recruits.

On April 24, Antoinette Donnelly, who among many other things was the *Chicago Daily Tribune*'s beauty editor, screamed this headline: "ROBERTSON VS. MISS DONNELLY IN DUEL ON FAT!" Making a good thing even better, she announced that she had challenged Robertson to a contest within the contest. She would find 25 overweight *men* to compete against his women. "A fat chance he has," she wrote, and went on to mention that the good doctor had a rather well-upholstered frame himself. Indeed, she suggested that *he* join her class, but Robertson, at first, declined. Well, she said, there were fatter men than him, and those were the ones she really wanted. "Let me be surrounded by men who are fat. I will show the doctor that a woman is nature's sweet restorer. Enlist beneath my standard and become my standard," the beauty editor concluded.

Donnelly, 33, was a prolific and overworked writer, which may be why she failed to notice the sexual allusion she had made in the preceding sentence. In 1913, she had joined the paper as both its "Playtime" expert, answering questions about grown-up entertaining, and, under the pseudonym Doris Blake, its syndicated, daily advice-to-the-lovelorn columnist. She also wrote a column entitled "Was It You?" in which she exposed the annoying people she encountered, almost always women, who were "chatterboxes," or "crepe hangers," or "overweight, ridiculous vamps." Having completed a diet book called *How to Reduce: New Waistlines for Old* with William Evans's assistant, by 1920 she was also the paper's prestigious beauty editor. This was an important assignment. She replaced Lillian Russell, feminist and former singer, Broadway star, and girlfriend of "Diamond" Jim Brady. Russell was known for her enormous appetites for food and men and for her voluptuous, early 20th-century body, but she was now devoting most of her time to the war effort and campaigning for the nearly secured women's suffrage. Donnelly, who believed "the national feminine cry is not votes for women— but fatless figures for women," had other priorities.

The Robertson–Donnelly stunt was scheduled to last 7 weeks and would cost the paper almost nothing. Robertson, as health commissioner, wanted to increase public awareness of obesity as a serious health threat. As he put it, "the amount of food wasted in fat is worse than shocking. It's a menace." There would be no prize for the winning team, because, as the spin went, they were already getting "the best prize in the world." All the contestants, however, did get their pictures and names in the paper along with their weights, and that made them minor, if temporary, celebrities (precursors to today's reality-TV weight-loss stars). The group got invited to parties and was given tickets to the theater. When the contest was over, they even made some public appearances.

Donnelly's men stole the headlines because their leader wrote them. After 6 days: "FAT FADING AS OBESE MEN GET DOWN TO WORK." After 18: "FAT MEN LOSE EIGHT POUNDS EACH IN TWO WEEKS."

The meal plans were printed daily so those not fortunate enough to be on a team could play along at home. On April 28, Robertson allowed his women an apple, two slices of bacon, a slice of bread with a teaspoon of butter, and coffee with skim milk for breakfast; clear soup, salad, and fruit for lunch; and any lean meat other than pork, string beans, graham bread with a teaspoon of butter, shredded cabbage with vinegar, and stewed fruit for dinner. Donnelly's menu was sparser: For breakfast, a baked apple or stewed prunes without sugar, one thin slice of rye bread without butter, two poached or soft-boiled eggs, and coffee without sugar. Lunch was vegetable soup and three crackers. Dinner was one portion of beef, lamb, or fowl; any vegetables except peas, potatoes, or beans; and one thin slice of rye bread without butter, followed by unsweetened black coffee, tea, or a glass of buttermilk.

Certain contestants began to stand out, and media favorites were established. Robertson's star pupil, Mrs. Frances Seeger of Berteau Avenue, lost 5 pounds fast and became the woman to beat. There was intrigue—Donnelly was informed that one of her class (no names named) had gone out and eaten a big dinner. Donnelly and Robertson did not have camera crews following the contestants around town, but they did have spies. The cheater wasn't thrown off the team; he was just given a serious warning that he would be if he lapsed again. In midcontest, Robertson decided that he *did* want to personally follow Donnelly's methods. Could his interest be genuine, or was he attempting to infiltrate "enemy" lines?

When it was over, more than 500 pounds had been lost; Frances Seeger had disappointed by finishing in eighth place; and only 12 of Robertson's pupils remained. Donnelly's men were victorious, beating the women by an average of 2.3 pounds. In addition, 20 stayed with the program, and a man was Chicago's biggest overall loser, beating the leading female by a pound. Donnelly was jubilant.

Soon afterward, Robertson and Donnelly began to receive requests from all over the country for advice about the best ways to reduce. "It seems that everyone is interested in the anti-fat movement," said Donnelly, "and so they should be." In October of 1921, she traveled to New York City. The health commissioner of New York had chosen "fifty fat men" and "fifty fat women" for a new biggest-loser event, this one sponsored by the *Chicago Daily Tribune*'s sister paper, the *New York Daily News*. Following the announcement, so many applicants mobbed the newspaper's offices that police had to be called in to prevent a riot.

THE WAR ON FAT

For a trend to catch on, different streams have to flow together. World War I wasn't the only catalyst for obesity intolerance. The women's movement, which began to coalesce in the 1870s and grew more powerful with each decade, won its first major victory when the 19th Amendment was ratified on August 18, 1920, and the granddaughters of the first suffragettes were born having the right to vote at legal age. Women had been making small inroads toward independence and power for years, attending colleges and graduate schools to study medicine, science, home economics, the liberal arts, business, and accounting. And yet that education meant nothing when it came time to decide public policy. Getting the vote symbolized a fresh beginning and a new world.

Girls bobbed their hair. Clothes got tighter and skirts got shorter. The overt sexiness of the so-called flapper was the new ideal. Many middle- and upper-class women attempted this air of chic insouciance, typified by unbuckled "flapping" rubber galoshes, cigarettes, and alcohol. ("Flasks are in every pocket, intoxication—if not too advanced a stage—counts not at all against one," proclaimed *Vogue*.) As automobiles became less expensive, college men and women got cars and the freedom they brought. There was Prohibition, but its restrictions were easily resolved with money, and most people who wanted jobs had them. The slender, cigarette-smoking, alcohol-drinking, short-skirted, lipstick-and-rouge-wearing girl of the jazz age would have been labeled something very unpleasant a generation before. Now, she was "it," the girl to be. Too much weight was just plain unfashionable, and it was cruelly mocked.

This desire to be slim led to the beginning of an American fad diet craze that would, ironically, escalate during the Great Depression. On May 20, 1925, a *Los Angeles Times* headline read "Students' Diets Menace Health" in reference to the "crazy dieting" going on at the University of Michigan, which included a very popular pineapple and lamb chop combination that was also the diet of choice at Smith College. College women dieting was a direct contrast to the attitude of their predecessors, who had perceived excess weight as a sign of health. It had been considered imperative that they look healthy. Early critics of higher education for women had stressed that too much learning would destroy the female reproductive system and cause sterility, a theory that, amazingly, went unchallenged. Archived letters from Smith women prior to 1920 often mentioned the need to gain weight, and a lot of it.

In 1925, the *Atlanta Constitution* listed the diets of various society ladies, all of whom were restricted to eating from one or two food groups: Spinach and only spinach, potatoes and milk, just fruits, and, naturally, pineapples and lamb chops. In her column, in an entry called "Freak Reducing Diets," Lulu Hunt Peters was the voice of reason, explaining that fad diets allowed about 800 calories a day, so weight was lost for as long as you could stand to be on one of them, which wouldn't be long. That's why people reduced on the pineapple and lamb chop diet, she said, not because of the diet's claim that the pineapple juice "digested" the lamb chop and prevented it from being stored in the body as fat.

In the same year Peters proposed an obesity tax, emphatically stating in a speech before the League of American Pen Women that "millions of fat people would start to reduce and make a scientific study of dieting which would result in better health for the entire nation" if they were financially penalized for eating too much.

In 1930, historian Eunice Fuller Barnard wrote in the *New York Times*: "It is too little recognized—and indeed may not be, fully, until the social and biological history of the twentieth century comes to be written—that it was our generation that precipitated the rapid change in diet." Wistfully, she remembered that just 20 years before, extra pounds had been a sign of good nature or good health, but now they had become an error in judgment. Barnard longed for the day when reducing meant just eating less candy or fewer potatoes. Now, eating was a science, and times were changing for the "professional" dieter.

Henry Ford, at age 66 still a frequent visitor to the San, had scientists working in nearby Dearborn, Michigan, to overcome what he called the "eating problem" of acidosis, which was the imaginary result of a system out of balance. In the midst of the greatest depression the country had ever known, Ford was concerned that the days of meat and potatoes had to come to an end. It had to be fruit for breakfast, protein for lunch, and carbohydrates for dinner. Ford's new belief was that longevity resulted from having an active mind, exercising, and eating food in the correct combinations. He planned to live to be 100.

THE SUDBURY SCHOOL FOR BOYS

In 1930, Henry Ford began an experiment. Some of the fortune he had acquired from the Model T, a car for people of limited means, would be used to finance a school for boys of limited means. They would be taught how to eat and live, according to Ford, and hopefully would graduate to the Ford Trade School in Detroit, where they would learn a vocation and someday work for the Ford Motor Company. The 31 boys between the ages of 13 and 17 were allowed no sugar, spices, cocoa, coffee, or tea. Salt was not permitted at the table. This would all be like dinnertime at the San, except that meat was included in the diet as long as it was eaten separately from carbohydrates and at the second meal of the day. (Lulu Hunt Peters, if she had had the opportunity, would likely have pointed

35

out the absurdity of this new way of eating. But Peters had become ill while traveling on the steamship *Adriatic* to a medical conference in London and died of pneumonia on June 27, 1930, at the age of 57.)

The school was a pastoral vision. The boys lived on a 3,000-acre, 18th-century farm in Sudbury, Massachusetts—the formerly deteriorating Wayside Inn—a place of such great beauty that it had once been praised by writers Nathaniel Hawthorne and Henry Wadsworth Longfellow, and had then been meticulously restored by Ford. Bread was baked from local whole wheat flour that had been ground at a local gristmill, and almost all of the produce was grown on the farm by the boys, who tended the sheep, cared for the chickens, and picked the apples and quince. It was an idyllic cult for a few handpicked wards of the state, and one more toy for an egomaniacal aging man who wanted to live forever. It was also an affirmation of yet another strange way of approaching dinner, that of making wonderful food less pleasurable. Widely known then as the Hay Diet, food combining would reemerge in the weight-loss-obsessed 1980s and never completely go away again.

THE MYSTERY OF WEIGHT LOSS

Vitalism, a philosophy that originated with chemists in the 15th century and gained popularity in the 19th century as science began to flourish, has been used to explain the mystery of weight loss. Defined as "a doctrine that the processes of life are not explicable by the laws of physics and chemistry alone and that life is in some part self-determining," it is perhaps somewhat easier to swallow than a directive to eat less and exercise more. It also clarifies the seemingly impossible: that just a few extra calories a day can add up, 10 years later, to obesity.

PART TWO

YOU'RE PERFECT;

NOW DIET!

3

PROHIBITION, DEPRESSION, AND BANANA CREAM PIE

ALTHOUGH IT WOULD SEEM LOGICAL THAT THE GREAT DEPRESSION MIGHT PUT A MORA-
torium on weight loss—or at least replace the fantasy ideal of the skinny
flapper—bizarre weight-loss schemes abounded in the 1930s. Lulu Hunt
Peters's strong voice of reason was gone without an immediate replacement. Nutrition experts were beginning to link obesity and early death,
and suddenly it was considered not only unattractive to be plump, but
dangerous as well. At the same time, scientists placed the blame of excess
weight directly on the individual by taking away all of the pre-1930s medical excuses, such as "glandular conditions." If you were overweight, it was
simply because you ate too much.

The American diet was shifting. Meat consumption was lower in the
1930s than it had been at any time since the USDA began tracking the
data, and wheat usage had likewise decreased. Sugar intake, however,
was on the rise. The 18th Amendment, in effect from 1919 through 1933,
prohibited the sale of alcohol in a country where many depended upon
it for business and pleasure. Although obtaining bootleg booze was possible (the first chapter of Irma S. Rombauer's self-published 1931 cookbook, *The Joy of Cooking*, begins, "Most cocktails containing liquor are
made today with gin and ingenuity"), it was expensive, and difficult to

39

come by unless you were in a large city. In the absence of a quick alcohol fix, Americans turned to sugar. As early as 1919, US food administrator Herbert Hoover testified before a subcommittee of the US House of Representatives, warning, "prohibition had had the effect of increasing the consumption of candy and sweet drinks to such an extent that a minor shortage in sugar existed." In 1920, the Federal Trade Commission on Sugar Supply and Prices, appointed by the US House of Representatives to investigate the shortages and sky-high prices asked for the household staple despite record supplies, blamed Prohibition for the greatly increased numbers of candy stores, ice cream parlors, and soft drink manufacturers. The Volstead Act, a law passed in 1919 that enabled the government to enforce the 18th Amendment, resulted in numerous unintended consequences, and a tremendous increase in sugar consumption was one of them.

AMERICA'S NATIONAL DRINK

There is something quintessentially American about cola. It's every man, woman, and child's beverage—the great equalizer. As early as 1891 *Harper's Weekly* had labeled it our "national drink," adding, "The millionaire may drink champagne while the poor man drinks beer, but they both drink soda water," so named because bicarbonate of soda created the bubbles.

John Pemberton developed Coca-Cola in the late 19th century as an alcohol-free beverage for the temperate times he envisioned, and it remains America in a glass in spite of its many competitors and imitators. As Tom Standage describes in *A History of the World in 6 Glasses*, Pemberton, an Atlanta pharmacist and experienced patent-medicine maker, was visionary enough to imagine a country that might someday require a substitute for hard liquor. To that end he combined coca leaves, kola nuts, and sugar into flavoring syrup for soda water. Coca and kola were popular ingredients in a number of quack remedies at the time, and they were advertised as being cures for just about anything. Coca leaves, when chewed, would release cocaine in miniscule but undoubtedly pleasant amounts, and kola nuts contained caffeine.

Thus, the original formula was a stimulating mix of sugar, caffeine, and cocaine, although any rush from the cocaine had to have been minimal or nonexistent. It was removed from the recipe in the early 20th century, which was fortuitous because food reformer Harvey Wiley, suspecting the beverage was detrimental to children, began investigating the formula. In 1911 he took the Coca-Cola Company to court, and after a long trial that was appealed and ultimately settled out of court, the company agreed to cut the amount of caffeine in the formula in half.

Around this time, Coca-Cola was becoming widely available. The drink was poured into the now-iconic 6-ounce, shapely, capped glass bottles. Coke was sold in grocery stores and at sporting events, and most people loved the taste. The drink had, and still has, about 13 calories per ounce, so although early calorie counters like Lulu Hunt Peters advised against it, a whole bottle was only a sweet 78-calorie misdemeanor. Its popularity did indeed grow during Prohibition, and at 5 cents a bottle, Coke was an affordable treat throughout the Depression. It replaced coffee and tea for some and alcohol for others, and it could be acceptably consumed, day and night, by everyone in the family. Long after both Prohibition and the Depression ended, the country's love affair with Coca-Cola endured.

TWICE AS MUCH FOR A NICKEL, TOO

In the 1930s, Pepsi-Cola was a struggling brand when Charles Guth, president of the Loft Candy Company and the cola's new owner, decided to sell 12-ounce bottles of Pepsi for 5 cents, the price for only 6 ounces of Coke. It was an inspired strategy. The additional cola and larger bottle cost Guth very little and bought him significant market share. In 1935 a person who said "Pepsi, please" was about to drink twice the number of calories in a bottle of Coca-Cola and probably not even know it. There was competition, friction, and litigation between Pepsi-Cola and Coca-Cola in the 1930s, but ultimately there was room in the soda market for both rivals, as people became accustomed to occasionally having a treat of a sweet beverage with fried and salty foods.

BUT WHAT'S FOR DESSERT?

In the early 1930s, new and extremely popular "all you can eat" restaurants were opening in major cities. If you were going to eat out, splurging on a meal that could cost anywhere between 60 cents and $1, value was a necessity and there had better be dessert. Restaurateurs reported that few customers ate more than one entree (that would seem gluttonous!), but many would order an éclair, ice cream, banana cream pie, and fresh fruit to finish off the meal. Eating all the sweets you wanted was acceptable, and the variety was astonishing. New York City hot spots began to specialize in one dessert variety or another to reel in diners who had sweet tooths—one eatery offered homey, comforting pies, puddings, and cakes; another hired a pastry chef to "devise elaborate patisseries" and offer exotic sweets. By 1931, Americans were consuming 105 pounds of sugar per capita a year. In 1919, the Federal Trade Commission had put the figure at 86.9 pounds. Eunice Fuller Barnard suggested that the nursery rhyme about little girls should be changed to "Sugar and spice and all things nice / That's what *Americans* are made of."

NOT ENOUGH SUGAR, AND TOO MUCH WHEAT

In 1931, American farmers were drowning in surplus wheat. The toaster had been invented in 1924 and sliced bread in 1928, but Americans were eating 143 pounds less wheat per capita than they had 40 years before. The surplus was due in part to some of the new fad diets, but it was also attributable to the poor economy, record harvests in Europe, and overproduction with little thought given to levels of supply and demand. Still, much of the blame was placed on women and their desire to "reduce." To that point, William J. Spillman, former chief of the Office of Farm Management, agreed that bread was fattening, but added, "It might be a good idea for our wheat friends to take a leaf out of the propaganda book of the cigarette folks . . . and organize a counterpropaganda of their own." Science writer Carl Malmberg thought it ironic that a perfectly good food like bread had so completely gone out of fashion among those who could still afford to eat whatever they desired. And although a calorie is a calorie when it comes to carbohydrates—there are 4 calories per gram whether they're in sugar or starch—there are a lot more of them lurking in an unlimited dessert buffet, ice cream, candy, and soft drinks.

CANDY IS DANDY

There was also a variety of new, processed foods drenched in sugary syrups from which to choose, and whether or not they were healthy choices was confusing. How could anyone really understand what was best to eat if someone as prestigious as Ruth Atwater, a former professor of home economics at the University of Chicago (and at that time director of marketing for the National Association of Canners) and daughter of the venerated Wilbur Olin Atwater, assured the public that commercially canned foods were not only identical in nutritional value to fresh foods, they were actually superior since the sugar in the syrup added more *energy*? This promotional propaganda was reported in the *Journal of Home Economics,* a publication that was edited by Ruth's sister Helen and funded by food processors. The information then made its way into various magazine articles and print ads.

"Pure" Karo table syrup ("rich in Dextrose, the food-energy sugar") was also advertised as a wholesome choice. "Of course we eat Karo!" say the five identical little Canadian girls famous throughout the world as the Dionne quintuplets in a 1935 ad for the corn syrup, which boasted the American Medical Association seal of approval. In 1937, Baby Ruth candy bars were advertised as the "delicious energizing" (rich in dextrose!) way to replenish energy. If food scientists and physicians said that energy was good for you, didn't that mean that all calories were good for you?

MOTHER'S MEALTIME HELPERS

Food processing was beginning to homogenize the American diet. There were (and of course still are) popular regional dishes; more lobster was eaten in Maine than Iowa, and more pecan pie in Georgia than New

Jersey. But for those who considered cooking just one more domestic chore, packaged, processed, canned, and frozen foods promised to take the drudgery out of meal preparation, especially when tight budgets had eliminated household help for all but the wealthy. Experts like Ruth Atwater assured the housewife that she was doing the right thing for her family by serving meals prepared with these foods.

Consistency of product, along with devotion to nutrition, science, and technology, was shaping the perception of the American diet around the globe. When the first edition of *Larousse Gastronomique*, a monumental food encyclopedia edited by Frenchman Prosper Montagné, was published in 1938, the entry on American cooking references the standardizations based on the countrywide distribution of factory-produced foods. This mass production must have seemed unusual to a Frenchman who was devoted to his local cuisine. Montagné states incredulously that "food is advertised and sold quite as much for its food value as for its enjoyment," and goes on to observe, years before McDonald's served its first Happy Meal, that it is characteristic of Americans to eat as quickly as possible for as little money as possible. The great chef Auguste Escoffier died before *Larousse* was published, but not before he wrote the book's preface, which he begins with these words: "The history of the table of a nation is a reflection of the civilization of that nation." In other words, sit down for a meal in France and observe the best of French culture. It is unlikely that Escoffier or Montagné would have said the same about a meal in the United States.

We were, in fact, as civilized as most, but it was also true that our dietary history was becoming more dysfunctional by the decade, and it didn't take a Frenchman to figure this out. "Only in the last two decades, and mainly in America, has a dish fit one year to set before a King been regarded in the next as a mess of more or less unhealthy pottage, and vice versa," Eunice Fuller Barnard wrote in 1930, commenting on the recommendations of home economists that seemed to change by the hour. The American attitude toward food was becoming unique in its paradoxical devotion to science, business, health, convenience, and weight-loss methods that were most peculiar.

44

KEEPING IT SIMPLE

Viral marketing materials of the time often came in the form of mass-distributed pamphlets directed at the housewife who wanted to keep her family healthy and her husband successful while she stayed trim. The California Fruit Growers Exchange produced quite a few of these, such as *Telling Fortunes with Foods,* a 1929 booklet recommending Sunkist oranges and lemons for everything from treating the fictitious disease acidosis to relieving fatigue, and, naturally, for weight loss. If a woman didn't serve oranges, terrible things would happen. Her husband would lose his edge in the boardroom, and she would lose her edge in the bedroom.

Many of the new fad diets originated from these heavily advertised and well-marketed schemes promoting particular foods. For example, the Hollywood 18-Day Diet, another idea promoted by the California Fruit Growers Exchange, allowed a meager 585 calories a day of grapefruit, orange, melba toast, raw vegetables, hard-boiled eggs, and black coffee. While the unemployed waited in breadlines and the working poor had a typical budget of $8 a week to feed a family of four, many middle- and upper-middle-class Americans returned by choice to the asceticism of dietary deprivation.

TAKING BACK CONTROL

When you feel that things are out of your control, it is natural to grasp for control of *something.* During the Great Depression, when even if there was enough today there might not be enough tomorrow, you could nag your spouse and scold your children, or you could begin one of the oddly limiting diets to give structure to your life. You might gain a temporary sense of calm from knowing that you could eat only citrus fruits and melba toast, as well as a sense of accomplishment when you lost a few pounds. During hard times, countrywide or individual, that sense of accomplishment, pride, and self-control often was the goal. Lose, regain, and then optimistically pick yourself up, dust yourself off, and start all over again. Losing weight by means of a fad diet became a fad in itself.

In 1935, when Carl Malmberg published an exposé of these senseless

45

fad diets, he realistically stated: "The premise that most people eat more than is good for them . . . might have had just a germ of truth in it back in the days when a chicken was supposed to be stewing in every pot, but now, with the seventh lean year of the depression almost upon us, it must be dismissed as pure nonsense." He added that "no single subject, with the probable exception of religion, has had grow around it a larger body of error, misinformation and just plain buncombe than the subject of diet."

THE HAYWIRE DIET

Buncombe it may have been, but for many the method of choice was the Henry Ford–endorsed Hay Diet. William Howard Hay, MD, formerly a pun-loving hay fever specialist, formulated his "health plan" based on the premise that protein and carbohydrates could never, under any circumstances, be eaten at the same meal. Sandwiches, of course, were forbidden. Syndicated medical columnist Logan Clendening, MD, condemned the diet and wrote, "more food notions flourish in the United States than any other civilized country." He was clearly exasperated by a population that seemed "profoundly ignorant" of the most elementary facts about nutrition. Ida Jean Kain, a dietitian who had once worked for John Harvey Kellogg and was now the syndicated health and nutrition columnist for the *Washington Post,* agreed. She called the diet "haywire," reminding readers that for goodness sake even a *potato* contains protein. Malmberg predicted the Atkins low-carb versus Pritikin low-fat wars by decades, saying: "It is only a matter of time until we shall hear the battle between the starches and proteins dramatized and fought out on the radio."

Clendening and Ida Jean Kain may have been scientists, but Hay was one of the most highly regarded nutritionists in the country, and also a licensed physician. To further confound things, much of what Hay advocated was sensible: eating nourishing foods sparingly, and only when hungry. There is good advice along with his steadfast rule. So how did the average American know whom to believe?

Hay's bizarre diet wasn't the only one to receive medical approval. A plan involving bananas and skim milk was endorsed by two doctors: Dr.

G. A. Harrop Jr. of Johns Hopkins University in Baltimore and Dr. Herman N. Bundesen, president of the Chicago Board of Health. Bundesen used a test group of three young women, who lost a combined 32 pounds in 30 days, proving, he said, that "dieting to reduce is practical, easy, and healthful." The United Fruit Company outlined all of the essentials of this diet in a (very) little booklet showing the American Medical Association seal of approval on its cover. The plan? For the first 10 to 14 days, eat 4 to 6 bananas, drink 3 or 4 glasses of skim milk, and have a small amount of vegetables. For the next 10 to 14 days, add some meat, eggs, or fish. While following this plan for up to 28 days, therefore, dieters existed on about 1,200 calories or less per day. Anyone following this calorie-restricted plan would undoubtedly lose weight—and gain it back as soon as he or she went back to a normal diet.

This was one of many food-group-specific diets to choose from—raw tomatoes and hard-boiled eggs, baked potatoes and buttermilk. Paul Whiteman, a famous bandleader of the era, ate only apples until he switched to pineapple and lamb chops. He lost so much weight that the love of his life agreed to marry him, at least according to Antoinette Donnelly.

Welch's Grape Juice ran print ads in every major paper in the country featuring 43-year-old entertainer Irene Rich, who still weighed the same as she had when she was 16, thanks, she claimed, to drinking a glass of grape juice three times a day. Eventually even Ida Jean Kain joined the party. Her popular syndicated column—"Your Figure, Madame!"—recommends thoroughly and depressingly chewing half a head of iceberg lettuce tossed with mineral-oil-based "Reducer's French Dressing" before every meal. Food, she predicts, will be unappealing following the bland and difficult to eat salad, and you will reduce by up to 2 pounds a week.

There was comfort in knowing exactly what to do, for as long as you could stand eating just bananas or chewing your way through a head of iceberg lettuce every day. After that, there were ice cream and chocolate cake. Losing weight to regain it to lose it again, or yo-yo dieting, was becoming part of the American way of life.

But if dieting seemed too difficult, perhaps there was an easier way.

4

DEATH BY DINITROPHENOL

IT WAS EXTRAORDINARY, BUT TRUE. MEN WORKING IN A NEW JERSEY EXPLOSIVES manufacturing plant were losing weight for no apparent reason. Researchers, including chemists at Stanford University, looked into the strange phenomenon. In 1933, the *Journal of the American Medical Association* published the Stanford study, and it seemed miraculous. Dinitrophenol, a benzene derivative used in the manufacture of explosives such as TNT, could cause weight loss without eating less or exercising more. When it was administered to 35 obese patients, they all lost weight effortlessly. Although the unsuspecting factory workers had inhaled the miracle substance from the air and absorbed it through their skin, the Stanford subjects were administered dinitrophenol in pill form. America had its first "fat burner."

That's what dinitrophenol did. It burned fat by increasing a person's base rate of metabolism by two to eight times. The user became warm, even feverish, and broke out in a sweat. This increase in body heat worked so well that it had been used to keep inadequately clothed Russian soldiers warm during World War I. There were some other "minor" side effects, like a change in the ability to taste. Turning yellow was also a possibility; that was not surprising because the chemical was used to dye textiles. William Brady, the physician who had replaced the late Lulu Hunt Peters and wrote the "Personal Health Service" column for the *Los Angeles Times*, claimed to be using it and said he didn't mind the side effects because he was effortlessly losing so much weight. The results were so extraordinary that even the conservative expert in preventive medicine, William Evans of Chicago, had to admit that it was the most effective means of weight loss ever developed. He recommended it to his readers, but only under the supervision of a physician, because, he said, "it is dangerous and it may cause death, and there is no way of knowing in advance if it will harm a given person." By June 1934, Brady was no longer so sure about the drug. His headline read: "The New Reduction Medicine Kills a Person Here and There," referring to a young woman who had died after taking 16 capsules of dinitrophenol in 5 days. Earlier that month, Emory University scientists had said that it might destroy white corpuscles and cause "almost certain death." Those World War I soldiers, it turned out, had been playing Russian roulette.

W. G. Campbell, head of the FDA, warned that dinitrophenol could cause "profound disturbances" and should not be used by anyone suffering from heart, liver, or kidney disease. In 1935, 12 women in the San Francisco Bay area who had been using it for weight loss were temporarily blinded as a result of cataract formation induced by dinitrophenol. The following year, the same thing happened to 100 people in Los Angeles. Some underwent surgery to restore their vision. Two Cleveland physicians reported that dinitrophenol was a possible cause of heart disease. New York doctors claimed it might cause congenital deformities. The problem was, it was an easily available over-the-counter drug marketed under numerous names like Nitromet, Nitra-phen, Redusols, and Formula 281, but you could also buy it as just plain Slim.

In 1938, a new law was passed that allowed the Federal Trade Commission (FTC) to pull a product from the shelves if it was falsely advertised and considered dangerous. The first thing the FTC did after that law was passed was to obtain a restraining order against the Hartman drug chain of Chicago, preventing sales of Formula 281. The order was based on an advertisement that stated that the pill helped reduce weight, was "widely prescribed by physicians," and had been used successfully for 4 years. Dinitrophenol became available by prescription only. Many people were still willing to gamble that they would be unaffected, and most were correct. The new advertising slogan could have been: "If it doesn't kill you, you'll lose weight." It's available online even today.

SHED POUNDS WITH SPEED

Benzedrine, an amphetamine developed in 1932 as a nasal inhalant for the relief of asthma (and quickly discovered by college kids cramming for finals), was promoted at the end of the decade as a miracle drug to cure fatigue, depression, impotence, and—yes—obesity. Dexedrine (dextroamphetamine) and many others soon followed. Despite a 1943 warning against the use of amphetamines issued by the American Medical Association, physicians nevertheless continued to prescribe them freely for weight loss, often with barbiturates on the side to calm the inevitable nervous reaction to what later came to be known as speed. Drug companies found themselves in a race to produce the best and longest-lasting amphetamine. This was, in part, a result of 180,000,000 pills that were handed out to sleep-deprived troops during World War II; many GIs kept up the habit when they returned home. In 1952, nearly 3 billion 60-milligram tablets were being produced annually, and, although Benzedrine also became available by prescription only in 1959, by 1970 the number had ballooned to 8 billion, and the *Wall Street Journal* estimated that 8 percent of *all* prescriptions were being written for amphetamines, primarily for weight loss. And women weren't the only ones asking their doctors for these drugs. American men now had a diet product they could feel comfortable using, a masculine pill that allowed truckers to drive all night and swingers to make love 'til dawn.

In addition to this new variety of weight-loss pills, various topical creams also became available at drugstores, such as the subtly named Fatoff and Slendaform. Another, Marmola, was made of dried animal thyroid gland and seaweed as well as dangerous cathartics. "Like all thyroid preparations," warned *Time* magazine, "Marmola may cause a user to drop dead." And of course, there were also the mixes such as Dr. Stoll's Diet Aid, which contained cornstarch, sugar, cocoa powder, and caramel. You mixed a spoonful of the stuff into hot water as a meal replacement for breakfast and lunch; it was the first of the many liquid diets of the future.

By the mid-1930s, weight loss had become an established American industry. Others may have worried about feeding their families, but if you had enough to eat during the Depression, you might well have starved yourself instead, because dieting was the thing to do. If you did, you were trendy, chic, sophisticated, and informed about the latest scientific breakthroughs. It was as if the Wizard of Oz himself had come to town, concocting phony weight-loss schemes that everyone believed in whether they worked or not, because they believed in him.

And then in 1939 we, as a nation, became distracted by larger, looming issues. Women who had recently existed by choice on bananas and skim milk would soon deal with rationing, the strain of having husbands and sons fighting overseas, full-time jobs, and trying to cobble together dinner fast and without enough of the usual staples. Dieting as a hobby temporarily lost its appeal.

5

WEIGHT-LOSS MORATORIUM

"HAPPY DAYS ARE HERE AGAIN" WAS THE THEME SONG OF FRANKLIN DELANO ROOS-evelt's 1932 presidential campaign. In spite of a brief recession in 1937, the sentiment was no longer hyperbole by 1940. The reality, of course, was that times were better because of the war in Europe, and some feared that the improved economy was neither real nor sustainable. "Despite myriad uncertainties," columnist H. J. Nelson assured in *Barron's*, "the pace of business in the United States continues strong. The *Barron's* business index that ended December 23, 1939, was the highest since May 1930." The *Wall Street Journal* predicted that 1940 would be one of the best years in history for the automotive industry, and a *New York Times* survey of major department store presidents indicated that retailers were optimistic.

People were once again traveling by rail, air, and bus as passenger lists swelled to pre-Depression-era numbers. Manufacturing, too, saw increased production, as steel, lumber, cement, and coal plants struggled to keep pace with demand for materials needed to build overseas military bases, airfields, and highways. The American food supply was in surplus. There was even talk of a shortage of skilled labor on the horizon.

But the good times came to an abrupt end on December 7, 1941, when Japanese planes attacked Pearl Harbor. Shortly after this first attack on US soil, America declared war on Japan.

FEEDING THE FREE WORLD

The requirements of feeding our troops and allies and of meeting the needs of the Red Cross in attempting to feed starving European citizens were staggering. Britain, whose 1941 civilian food consumption dropped to 37 percent less than normal, required 200,000 tons of US food a month, including evaporated milk, cheeses, dried fruits, dried beans, and pork. Growing food on any patch of land you had access to—your front yard, a community park, or a vacant lot—became both patriotic and necessary as the US and UK governments alike urged citizens to plant victory gardens. These small gardens cumulatively yielded a large harvest that was used as an emergency food supply and for school lunches, as well as giving the gardeners an inexpensive, varied diet with numerous fresh (not canned) vegetables. It was a wildly successful program, and by the end of 1943, 20 million victory gardens were producing 40 percent of America's vegetables.

All of this fresh produce resulted in the government urging a return to canning, which made a temporary, if brief, comeback, as housewives who had never before preserved fruits and vegetables complained of exploding jars, ruined stoves, and food poisoning. Still, women were urged to transport themselves back in time. The "old-fashioned housekeeping methods for the housewife of today, who not only refuses to bake her own bread, but also refuses to cut it" was strongly recommended by a scolding *New York Times* reporter (referencing, of course, the ubiquitous sliced, mass-produced white bread that now lined grocery store shelves). For the lady of the house, stoicism and personal sacrifice were ways she could support her country.

HONEY, THEY SHRUNK THE PANTRY

The hoarding of clothing and food began almost immediately after the declaration of war. In the first months of 1942, America experienced the highest retail sales in its history as people rushed to stock up on absolutely anything they feared would become scarce. There were already government controls in place on wool, tin, and rubber, and rumors were circulating that sugar rationing would begin in May. This was ironic because just a few months before, during the sugar surplus summer of 1941, it had been considered unpatriotic to take less than 3 teaspoons in your coffee, whether you wanted them or not.

Our soldiers were referred to as "the best-fed army in history," and they were. But as far as most of the country was concerned, the personal sacrifice necessary to keep them that way while simultaneously feeding half of Europe had lost its charm. There was no longer an easy willingness to "tighten the belt" as there had been during World War I. Whether it was due to the recent impact of the Depression, memories of World War I food shortages, or simply a love affair with sweet coffee, thousands mobbed grocery stores demanding the biggest bags of sugar available, 100 pounds if they could get their arms around them. The new rationing booklets issued in May 1942 allowed $\frac{1}{2}$ pound of sugar per person per week, with a household limit of 2 pounds per person. Thus, a family of four could have 8 pounds of sugar in the cupboard at any given time —hardly a negligible amount. But still, Americans panicked. Canned foods, condensed milk, and coffee were also hoarded. The country that had only recently become reacquainted with abundance was reluctant to let go of those comforts. It wasn't just about the soldiers anymore—American citizens were supposed to be the best-fed people in the world.

AMERICA LEARNS HOW TO EAT

In looking at the brighter side of rationing, many magazine and newspaper articles stressed that these restrictions would probably improve the American diet. "In the pre-ration era we did not bother much about nutrition. Now we face its challenge," wrote Cornell University professor of nutrition Clive M. McCay in 1943, adding, "Thousands of Americans have gone to premature graves from overeating and keeping their bodies too fat." Now, he continued, housewives would have to learn how to get the most nutritional value for their ration-book dollar. Similar to Wilbur Atwater and his disciples of decades before, McCay considered eating to be no more than a way to fuel the engine. The difference was that he had a lot of new information about what type of fuel was best. It wasn't just about the number of calories anymore, although he believed that a 150-pound male needed about 3,000 of them every day. Instead, it was also about his need for protein (70 grams), calcium (0.8 gram), vitamin C (75 milligrams), niacin (18 milligrams), and other vitamins and minerals that are required daily, all prescribed by McCay in difficult to comprehend amounts. Now that choices were limited, education was mandatory if you wanted to do right by your family.

Doing the right thing was becoming bewilderingly difficult without help. Eleven vitamins had been identified by then, but few people understood what they were or how to incorporate them into their diets. Consequently, almost one-third of Americans families were using vitamin supplements and eating vitamin-enriched foods, like white bread that was "enriched" by putting back some, but not all, of the B vitamins that had been removed during the processing of the wheat. Though there was no evidence that synthetic vitamins had any nutritive benefit whatsoever, an industry had been born. It didn't much matter if there was proof of its benefits or not—most customers didn't know enough about nutrition to be discerning. A 1944 Gallup poll revealed that 80 percent of American housewives didn't know the difference between a vitamin and a calorie.

FOOD RATION DIET

Bengamin Gayelord Hauser promoted himself as a "famous Viennese health expert." He was German, actually, but Austria must have seemed preferable as a birthplace after the war. He *was* famous, for being the nutritionist of both Marlene Dietrich and Greta Garbo, although he was neither a medical doctor nor a nutritionist but a "naturopath." Handsome and with a talent for both marketing himself and writing like a tabloid gossip columnist, Hauser had developed a career in "health" with very few credentials. In the previous decade, as "a nationally known authority on food science," he had focused on weight loss. His plan centered on drinking a laxative called Swiss Kriss manufactured not in Switzerland, but in Milwaukee by Modern Health Products, a company that he co-owned. In addition to Swiss Kriss, his diet consisted of fruits, vegetables, brewer's yeast, yogurt, wheat germ, blackstrap molasses, powdered skim milk, and "vegetable salts," which were also manufactured by Modern Health Products. (The laxative, salts, and many other Hauser dietary supplements are still sold.)

Hauser was thrilled with rationing: "The last war taught us that gout and rheumatism disappeared with the disappearance of big busts, tummies, and hips." He predicted that limiting Americans' food intake could only improve their waistlines.

Food rationing was changing the American diet. The consumption of sugar, eggs, and butter decreased as women baked less due to food constraints and, more likely, time constraints. Data indicated that people ate fewer fresh fruits and vegetables (with the notable exception of plentiful and cheap government-subsidized corn), but with so many victory gardens, this was difficult to quantify. They were consuming far less fish, in spite of the fact that fresh fish was not rationed. The consumption of poultry products, also not restricted, soared. About 250 cheeses, including Camembert, Brie, and Bel Paese, were excluded from rationing because few people wanted them anyway, an advantage for the more sophisticated palates. It is possible that in some families, restriction inspired a more adventurous diet, and perhaps a healthier one, but statistics don't indicate that this was anything more than a minority position.

Rationing was in effect wherever food was served—hotels, restaurants, hospitals, and jails all required ration books and appropriate points. Although the rules were fairly lenient—$\frac{1}{2}$ pound of butter (2 sticks) per person per week was permissible—"foodleggers," as the new post-Prohibition black marketers were called, became a popular alternative source of food in many major cities.

SHOPPING CART RACKETEERS

An unfortunate crime wave began in war-torn and food-deprived Great Britain, where citrus fruits had disappeared from grocery shelves along with lard, shredded wheat, canned salmon, and onions, and eggs were rationed at two per person per week. In the first 3 months of 1941, more than 5,000 people were convicted of crimes such as hijacking food trucks and slaughtering farmers' livestock and speeding away with the fresh meat. The stolen goods were sold on the black market—to retail merchants and "speakeasy"-style restaurants. By 1943, rationing and food shortages resulted in a strong black market emerging in the United States as well.

"Bootleggers were ethical businessmen compared with wartime foodleggers," New York City mayor Fiorello LaGuardia admonished listeners in his February 1943 radio broadcast. Despite the fact that it was against the law to purchase rationed food without the appropriate number of ration stamps, food racketeers were thriving. The government's recommendation that American citizens voluntarily cut back on meat consumption in 1942 (a campaign called Share the Meat) proved ineffective. In March of 1943, beef and pork stamps were added to the ration books, which in turn caused the black market business to soar. Americans were willing to pay the price; meat was even more valuable than money.

When the war ended in 1945, price controls and rationing remained in effect on better cuts of meat, and enraged farmers withheld their livestock from the market. It could be purchased only at illegally high prices, and it was. The *Chicago Daily Tribune* reported in April 1946 that foodleggers slaughtered animals in Canada and smuggled the meat across the border into America, then returned to Canada with truckloads of American cigarettes and liquor.

By July 1946, public outrage led the Office of Price Administration (OPA) to remove all price ceilings, and ranchers flooded the market with beef. The supply was great, but demand for meat in a postwar boom economy was even greater, and prices soared. In September, the OPA, fearing inflation, reinstated price controls, causing farmers to once again withhold livestock, and a new, if temporary, shortage cycle began. President Harry S. Truman, concerned about reelection in a country demanding roast beef and ham, dismantled the OPA in October 1946 and ended the price controls. The shortages of the previous years, however, resulted in a national hunger for meat, and lots of it. It may have helped transform us, in the decade that followed, into a country where an inexpensive hamburger was rarely far away.

THE WAR ENDS, THE SHORTAGES DON'T

When World War II officially ended on August 14, 1945, much of Europe was suffering from serious food shortages. It was estimated that the problem might be three times as big as the food insecurities that had followed World War I. Herbert Hoover—who once again had been appointed boss of the food supply, though this time it was for most of the Western world—reported that Norway, Holland, Belgium, Greece, Poland, Yugoslavia, and the Baltic States were all suffering badly. Although the government hadn't imposed rationing during World War I, Hoover's Food Administration statistics showed American per capita food consumption had actually been *lower* in the period from 1917 to 1919 (Food Will Win the War!) than it was from 1942 through 1944. Meat and cooking oil consumption, in particular, had increased, in spite of rationing. There had been a definite shift in the average American's sense of entitlement when it came to mealtime.

LADIES, CAN YOU SPARE 10 POUNDS?

A series of articles written by nutritionist Ida Jean Kain and syndicated by the *Washington Post* began to appear in newspapers across the country in January of 1946. They served collectively as a national wake-up call for American women to get in shape in order to get (or keep) husbands. "Six million G.I.'s will soon be home, you know!" Kain enthusiastically wrote. "Competition is rugged. For the first time in history there won't be enough men to go around," she warned. Kain advised her readers to begin her new 18-Day Slim-Down Diet and lose 10 pounds. She also suggested that while it was important to be attractive, women shouldn't be *too* pretty. Guys, she believed, are wary of gorgeous girls: "Often the glamour girl is self-centered and, maybe, a sad sack with the skillet." So in addition to losing those 10 pounds, it was also a good idea to brush up on your cooking skills before your soldier came home. After all, "[a] girl has to catch his eye before he is interested in finding out how she cooks." This time the pressure to diet was about more than just fitting into the latest fashions. There were limited supplies of meat, butter, sugar—and men!

Kain's 18-day diet was a nutritious but punishing 1,000-calories-a-day plan of lean proteins, vegetables, and fresh fruit. Since American women weren't, on average, overweight, losing 10 pounds probably wasn't medically necessary for most. But weight loss was, yet again, becoming seen as imperative if not actually needed. Within months, a new array of diet pills, laxatives, starvation diets, and slenderizing creams would be all the rage, and credentialed experts would, one more time, recommend avoiding them and simply eating less if you wanted to lose weight.

The pressure was on to be postwar perfect, and your body was as good a place to start as any. Marriage, children, secure cash flow, and a beautiful house in the suburbs might be the American dream, but if it was elusive—and it often was—the sense of failure could be overwhelming. And even if you were able to meet these goals, the realization that it was ephemeral (or worse, that it wasn't making you happy) could be devastating.

Losing weight could take your mind off all of that and bring a temporary sense of accomplishment, a calmness that came from knowing what to do about something, even if it was just lunch.

6

WHO NEEDS CARBS?

IN 1935, A TIME WHEN MANY WOMEN WERE BECOMING DISPLEASED WITH THEIR FIGURES and confused about what they should and shouldn't eat, author and civil rights activist Fannie Hurst honestly and openly discussed her disordered eating in a memoir titled *No Food with My Meals*.

Hurst, who was at the time the most financially successful female writer in America (even if critics labeled her a "sob sister" for her melodramatic, romantic stories), writes about her struggles with "neurosis, psychosis, and acidosis"—that is, her attempt to be slimmer than she was ever meant to be in an era that equated thinness with beauty and integrity. "It was about four years ago that the slimming phobia of my sex and era took hold," she begins, describing the passion for losing weight that swept the country during the Great Depression. Hurst remembers her idyllic childhood as the only daughter of an affluent St. Louis shoe manufacturer and his stylish wife, when every day began with a big midwestern breakfast set out by household staff. Oatmeal with plenty of butter, sugar, and cream; a platter of bacon and eggs; toast or hot biscuits wrapped in a red-and-white-checkered napkin and cradled in a wicker basket; hominy or grits or stacks of griddle cakes with apple jelly; and "coffee and plenty of it," served with warm coffee cake thickly sprinkled with cinnamon and sugar—the meal is similar to a special-occasion buffet a child might enjoy in a luxury hotel dining room today. "I was reared to like breakfast," Hurst says, adding that she hasn't eaten it in years.

This radical feminist who kept not only her own name after marriage but also her own apartment nevertheless pressures herself to conform to a contemporary ideal of beauty at a time when, she writes, "bust measurements of the potential and actual mothers of the race dropped to the proportions of their young sons and brothers." She lists some of the products she can buy to help shed pounds—enameled rolling pins for kneading flesh, reduction salts, rowing machines. New industries were born, she says, and "spas began to find obesity, real and imagined, more profitable than liver complaints, gallstones and gout all rolled into one."

As her short treatise comes to an end, Hurst becomes angry at the manipulative and capricious whims of a nation where the *Venus de Milo,* the *Mona Lisa,* and Lillian Russell are no longer standards of beauty and the last decade's ideal becomes this year's joke. She blames the "bizarre and little so-called civilization known as Hollywood, home of the eighteen day diet . . . and almost every reduction fad known to this tormented year of our Lord" for fueling the trend. (She had recently spent time in Hollywood while her best-selling novel *Imitation of Life* was being made into a motion picture, and she disliked the town intensely.) Hurst has been stringently dieting for so long that, she writes, "It remains practically impossible to sit down whole-heartedly to a meal . . . to violate by one calorie is to invite regrets out of all proportion to the delights of the transgression." These are the words of a woman nibbling around the edges of anorexia, and perhaps an inadvertent warning that a segment of the population is heading the same way.

THE FEMINIST AND THE EXPLORER

Fannie Hurst married concert pianist Jacques Danielson in 1915, but their marriage was kept secret from everyone except her parents and a few friends until an Associated Press reporter broke the story that became front-page news in May 1920. ("Novelist Reveals Her 5-Year Trial Marriage," read one headline, while another said, "Fannie Hurst Wed; Hid Secret 5 Years.") Hurst and Danielson maintained separate apartments in an attempt to "keep the dew on the rose," as she put it, adding, "Neither my husband nor I lives in Greenwich Village nor wears horn-rimmed spectacles. We believe in love but not Free Love."

Although they said they planned to continue living apart, the couple made it clear that the "trial" was over, and that this was "an announcement and not an annulment." They remained married until Danielson's death in 1952. "We had it nice," Hurst would frequently say after he died, giving their story a happy ending. Nevertheless, in 1922 she began an ongoing romantic affair with one of the most extraordinary men of her time: the charismatic writer, lecturer, and Arctic explorer Vilhjalmur Stefansson. In what could have been a Fannie Hurst plot, the (secretly married) Greenwich Village intellectual who was to inadvertently lay the foundation for every high-fat, low-carb diet of the century had captured the heart of the (now openly married) uptown dietary ascetic.

NOT BY BREAD ALONE

Stefansson was born in what is now Manitoba, Canada, in 1879. His Icelandic immigrant parents emigrated to North Dakota when he was 2 years old, where he grew up working on farms and herding cattle. After graduating from the University of Iowa, he entered the graduate program in divinity at Harvard University, but transferred to the department of anthropology a year later.

In 1906 he resigned his position as teaching fellow in anthropology at Harvard and went to the Arctic for the first of what would become 14 years of rarely interrupted ethnographic studies of the Inuit, combined with rigorous and sometimes solitary polar exploration. Perhaps because of his Icelandic heritage, he had a passionate love for the region, believing it majestically beautiful as well as eminently livable if approached correctly. Other polar explorers like Robert Peary and Ernest Shackleton avoided traveling during the coldest times of the year and kept themselves separate from the native population unless they needed a guide or a mistress. Stefansson learned to speak Inuktitut and lived with and as the Inuit did, hunting for all of his own food and eating a diet of meat, fish, and fat exclusively for years at a time. (By way of contrast, when Peary left New York City by ship in his quest to reach the North Pole in 1908, 16,000 pounds of flour and 40,000 pounds of corned beef accompanied him and his men.)

As an anthropologist, Stefansson became part of the culture he was studying—a distinctly different approach than that of his peers, who kept at a distance while observing and assessing "the other" from a decidedly superior point of view. This is not to say that he was without bigotry in his work. Although respectful of what he refers to as Eskimo culture, he consistently calls it "primitive" and, occasionally, "uncivilized." However, at a time when it was not unusual for human "living specimens" to be shipped halfway across the world and displayed as zoological curiosities, he had a more heightened sensibility than most.

Stefansson married an Inuit woman, Fanny Pannigabluk, whom he called Pan, and they had a son. Perhaps fearful of rampant racial prejudice—or perhaps for less noble reasons—he never brought his Inuit family to America. He left the Arctic in 1920, never to see them again (though he did continue to support them financially). He gave up on exploring, he said, because airplanes and dirigibles brought with them so much "ease, safety, comfort, and certainty of attainment" that discovery had become, for him, "more or less humdrum." His August 27, 1962, front-page *New York Times* obituary (that spilled over onto another page inside the paper) referred to him as "among the last of the dog team explorers."

In his Greenwich Village apartment in New York City, Stefansson lived very differently. There, he was the sophisticated celebrity bachelor, dining at bohemian restaurants with Amelia Earhart and Charles Lindberg, touring on a lucrative lecture circuit, and remaining "single" until Pan's death in 1940. This was his split-screen existence—husband, father, and Arctic explorer living a when-in-Nome lifestyle up north, and best-selling author, lecturer, and charming man-about-town involved with several women while in Manhattan.

Fannie Hurst, of course, was one of them—he was her lover for more than 17 years. They were both fascinated by food, but from very different perspectives. Her obsession was with what she *wouldn't* allow herself to eat, and it lasted a lifetime. Stefansson was interested in what he *did* eat, and, in particular, the fact that the Inuit diet kept him and his men strong under the harshest conditions. His Arctic diet was one that Wilbur Atwater, Lulu Hunt Peters, and William Evans would never have condoned. He wrote about what he had been *taught* to eat in a series of articles for *Harper's Monthly*:

63

It was desirable to eat fruits and vegetables, including nuts and coarse grains. The less meat you ate the better for you. If you ate a good deal of it, you would develop rheumatism, hardening of the arteries, and high blood pressure, with a tendency to breakdown of the kidneys—in short, premature old age. An extreme variant had it that you would live more healthy, happily, and longer if you became a vegetarian.

Specifically it was believed, when our field studies began, that without vegetables in your diet you would develop scurvy. It was a "known fact" that sailors, miners, and explorers frequently died of scurvy "because they did not have vegetables and fruits." This was long before Vitamin C was publicized.

Stefansson, who said he lived on only fish or meat for an aggregate of more than 5 years, set out to prove that the nutritionists were wrong, that man was perfectly capable of "living off the country"—and by this he meant eating only meat and fish—*especially* if the country was the frozen Arctic. There might be some diets as good (he mentions the vegetarian diet famously followed by George Bernard Shaw as an example), but there was no diet *better* than one that was comprised of fat and protein and virtually carbohydrate free. Everything the body required could be found in meat, fish, and bones, he believed.

Americans were consuming 40 to 60 fewer pounds of meat annually in the 1930s than in the 1830s, due in part to the horrors of the meat-packing industry as revealed by Upton Sinclair in his novel *The Jungle*, high beef prices in a depressed economy, changing tastes during World War I and Prohibition, and the advice of dietitians. Even with consumption in decline, however, most Americans still liked red meat and lots of it, and this was one of the things that made the research and writings of Vilhjalmur Stefansson so compelling.

He obtained a grant from the Institute of American Meat Packers (IAMP) to scientifically prove his theory that an all-meat diet was equal to or better than a balanced one and would not result in scurvy or calcium deficiency. He and a former colleague volunteered to be subjects in a study supervised by nutritionists, anthropologists, and physicians from the Russell Sage Institute of Pathology at Bellevue Hospital, the American Museum of Natural History, and Cornell University Medical College in New York City; Johns Hopkins University in Baltimore; the University of Chicago; and Harvard University. The IAMP, which had a physician on the committee as well, was given warning that the scientists "would lean backwards to make sure nothing in the results would ever be suspected of having been influenced by the money."

THE INUIT DIET

In 1930, when the results of the trial were presented, researchers described the 48-year-old Stefansson as single, well developed except for (surprisingly) soft and flabby muscles, and suffering from gingivitis. Subject number two, 38-year-old Karsten Anderson, a former Arctic explorer turned Florida citrus grower, was depicted as thin and well developed. He had once contracted scurvy when in the Arctic with Stefansson but was cured, he said, after eating raw meat. The third subject, a physician and nonexplorer, quit after 10 days.

Stefansson and Anderson ate only beef, lamb, veal, pork, chicken, liver, kidney, brain, heart, sweetbreads, bone marrow, bacon, and fat and drank only coffee, tea, broth, and water for a year. Their calories averaged 2,600 a day, and their macronutrient breakdown was 15 to 25 percent protein, 75 to 85 percent fat, and 1 to 2 percent carbohydrates from glycogen, a form of glucose stored in the livers and muscles of animals. The subjects were regularly tested for ketosis—a potentially dangerous condition that can occur when the liver converts fats into fatty acids and ketones, or incompletely burned fats, are flushed out of the body. Both men finished the year in good physical condition, and Stefansson was even cured of his gingivitis. Although they lost some weight in the first week, they quickly gained it back, and after that their weight remained relatively stable. In the end, Anderson had lost a few pounds and Stefansson, who had wanted to lose about 9 pounds, did. According to the authors of the study, "any loss of weight was due to diminished food intake." Stefansson's hypothesis was proven, at least for himself and Anderson, who both said they had never felt better in their lives.

BY MEAT ALONE

In the Arctic, where Stefansson and Anderson hunted and fished for their food, and even in 1930 New York City, where they didn't actually kill their own dinner, the meat the men ate wouldn't resemble what is readily available in most supermarkets today. All of the animal meat available to them was wild or naturally raised—in other words, "grass fed." They also consumed the entire animal or fish—they gnawed on the bones and devoured the livers, brains, kidneys, sweetbreads, hearts, and bone marrow. Indeed, Stefansson had once felt ill until his craving for calf's brain was satisfied. The organ meats and bones provided essential nutrients that kept them in good health, including sufficient vitamin C, which previously had been thought to be found only in fruits and vegetables. They consumed foods rich in vitamins and minerals.

Stefansson died in 1962. He had been teaching at Dartmouth College, as director of polar studies and curator of his own extensive library of the polar regions, since 1947. His papers are still housed there today, including diaries of his years as an explorer, photographs he took in the Arctic, and letters from Fannie Hurst. He had discovered and mapped some of the world's last major uncharted landmasses, envisioned the "great circle route" of airliners traveling from North America to Europe, worked with prominent American and Russian leaders in developing Biro-Bidjan as a refuge for Jews fleeing Eastern Europe in the 1930s (this autonomous Jewish state within Russia was, and still is, located in Siberia, and about 3,000 Jews currently make it their home), and wrote numerous books and articles on topics drawn from various fields of study, including anthropology, geopolitics, economics, linguistics, medicine, nutrition, and religion.

But it can be argued that Stefansson's most significant legacy was his impact on the diet and weight-loss industry. His two-subject experiment is still being used as "scientific proof" that high-fat diets result in weight loss and will do no harm. Though he couldn't have predicted the long-term implications of his words at the time, he became the grandfather of no- and low-carb diets and the muse of Robert Atkins, MD, when he wrote:

A phase of our experiment has a relation to slimming, slender-izing, reducing, the treatment of obesity. I was about ten pounds overweight at the beginning of the meat diet and lost all of it. This reminds me to say that Eskimos, when still on their native meats, are never corpulent—at least I have seen none. . . . See them striped [sic] and you do not find the abdominal protuberances and folds which are numerous at Coney Island beaches and so persuasive in arguments against nudism. There is no racial immunity among Eskimos to corpulence. You prove that by how quickly they get fat and how fat they grow on European diets.

In 1946 he wrote *Not by Bread Alone*, once again stating that he was only out to gather facts in a scientific manner, not to "prove" anything except the truth. He concluded once more that many diets were possible for optimal health and that the all-meat diet was just one of them.

In 1956, an "enlarged edition," now titled *The Fat of the Land*, was published, with commentaries by Fredrick Stare, PhD, MD, chairman of the department of nutrition at Harvard, and Paul Dudley White, MD, a Harvard cardiologist who became a household name as Dwight D. Eisenhower's personal physician and televised spokesperson following the president's heart attack. White, who had been a strong proponent of lessening the amount of fat in the American diet, conceded that "more controlled scientific data are needed by all concerned, especially by the high fat proponents."

THE MRS. SPRAT DIET

Alfred Pennington, MD, was a physician working for the industrial-medical division of E. I. du Pont de Nemours and Company in 1948, a time when the corporation was investigating the link between obesity and heart disease. He successfully tested a high-fat, high-protein, carbohydrate-restricted diet on himself and then on 20 male executives, including the chairman of the board. They lost an average of 22 pounds in 100 days, and he published his results in the trade journal *Industrial Medicine* in 1949.

67

Pennington had been a disciple of Blake Donaldson, MD, a physician who in the 1920s had prescribed a weight-loss diet of ½ pound of fatty meat three times a day, along with a "hotel portion" of ripe raw fruit or baked potato without salt; coffee or tea, water, and a half-hour walk before breakfast. Donaldson perfected his diet after having long discussions with Stefansson, whose work he credited. Stefansson later wrote that Donaldson had read about this diet in one of his earlier books, *The Friendly Arctic,* but thought that it would be more "acceptable" as a reducing diet if he altered it to include salad, fruit, and potatoes. Stefansson agreed that this would do no harm, reasoning that some "Eskimos" in Labrador and Alaska ate vegetables.

In 1950, *Holiday* magazine published a supplement about this revolutionary weight-loss theory based on Pennington's, Donaldson's, and Stefansson's findings. The cover called it the Eat-All-You-Want Reducing Diet, but the plan quickly became known as the Holiday Diet. Stefansson later said that it *should* have been called, chronologically, the Eskimo Diet, the Friendly Arctic Diet, the Blake Donaldson Diet, the Alfred W. Pennington Diet, the du Pont diet, and then, finally, the Holiday Diet, and he mentioned that he first published it in 1921 as a good all-around plan that could also be useful for reducing. He said that it had been a friendly collaboration, and that Donaldson had already thanked him personally for his influence on obesity research.

Holiday magazine attributed the great success of the topic to the fact that people actually enjoyed being on the plan, stating, "People welcomed a reducing diet that allowed them all they wanted of the food they liked so well, meat."

The high-fat, very-low-carb diet was now mainstream, and extremely popular for a short time. "Cholesterol" was becoming a household word in 1950, and after President Eisenhower suffered a heart attack, it became widely believed that fat, in particular, was to blame. "Everyone" knew that eating too much of it was dangerous. But even if this sequence of events hadn't occurred, it is doubtful that people would have stayed on the diet forever. Americans loved carbs as much as they loved meat. Maybe more.

PART THREE

HOW TO START AN EPIDEMIC

7

A PLAGUE IS BORN

THE AVERAGE LIFE SPAN IN 1950 WAS 67 YEARS, COMPARED TO 48 YEARS IN 1900.
Antibiotics and vaccinations had conquered most infectious diseases. Because bacteriological diseases were no longer commonplace, cardiovascular disease was now responsible for 56 percent of all deaths. The obese appeared to be at greater risk for heart disease, and thus, in postwar America, fat became the new enemy to fight.

"Americans are getting fat on too much food and too little work," proclaimed a 1950 article in the *New York Times*. Maude Behrman, the dietitian being quoted, went on to say that obesity was becoming a national problem.

It was thought to be a psychological problem, too; psychologists and doctors agreed that overeating was a consequence of being lazy and psychologically disturbed. The *New York Times* reported that in a paper published in the *Journal of the American Medical Association,* Massachusetts physician Dr. Max Millman wrote that obesity was a psychological problem caused by one or more of the following neuroses: a defense mechanism to prevent intimacy or avoid competition, excessive worrying, insecurity, an inferiority complex, or a need to "bolster importance" by being large. Psychiatrist Hilde Bruch, MD, believed that men equated "big" with intimidation. Women, said Dr. Bruch fancifully, became overweight to be neither male nor female, but a combination of both, and a mythological force. Another hypothesis was that women gained weight to replicate pregnancy, or to avoid it.

Within the decade, psychological profiles of the three most typical types of overeaters would be defined as 1) the aggressive eater who gains

71

weight to literally have more weight to throw around, 2) the passive and lonely eater who is comforted by food, and 3) the timid eater who is insulating himself from fear with additional padding.

A. D. Jonas, MD, stated somewhat similarly in *American Practitioner and Digest of Treatment*: "Many people overeat because they feel insecure, lack affection, are bored or have other emotional problems." Jonas was experimenting with methylcellulose, a synthetic appetite suppressant. Theoretically, when mixed with water and ingested, it would expand and create the illusion of being satiated. (It did, and although ineffective for weight loss, it is currently the active ingredient in a variety of laxatives.) Edward H. Rynearson, MD, of the Mayo Clinic in Rochester, Minnesota, speaking to a group of insurance-company medical men, insisted that an overweight person was nearly always a compulsive eater who turned to food the way an alcoholic turned to drink. He claimed that obesity was "the greatest single hazard to human life in the nation today," and that since there was an Alcoholics Anonymous, there should also be a Calories Anonymous. "There are not enough psychiatrists and psychoanalysts to treat all the nation's overeaters," he concluded. Harry J. Johnson, MD, director of the Life Extension Institute in New York, called obesity "the plague of the twentieth century."

All of this was quite amazing, because Americans were no heavier in 1950 than they had been in previous decades.

YOU'RE THE TOPS!

Although weight-loss support groups had been growing in popularity since Lulu Hunt Peters's World War I–era Watch Your Weight Anti-Kaiser clubs, the concept that obesity was an emotional problem that could be helped with therapy was novel.

The Metropolitan Life Insurance Company weight-loss charts, which had last been revised in 1942, were being recalculated to reflect the belief that people should weigh less. Group therapy, as recommended by Metropolitan Life, was a new way of getting there. Treating people in the company of others began as a novel approach to marriage counseling in the 1930s. After World War II, it became a necessity when there weren't enough trained therapists to deal with the multiple problems of returning soldiers. Now, it had evolved into a modern way to take off weight. Most of these groups were run by dietitians, not trained therapists, but they still often involved participants sharing their problems and fears.

In 1948, a Milwaukee woman named Esther Manz thought that she could bring the power of mutual support that she experienced in sessions preparing her for childbirth to her new challenge of losing weight. She and some friends formed TOPS: Take Off Pounds Sensibly. After an article about the group was published in a local newspaper, thousands of women contacted Manz about joining her club.

A TOPS meeting was comfortable, friendly, and fun. Chapters of TOPS, with names like Wimmin Slimmin and Classy Chassis, began to flourish all over the country. After reaching your desired weight, the goal was to maintain your weight loss for 3 months and then become one of the KOPS, an acronym for Keeps Off Pounds Sensibly. In those early days, a weekly meeting usually began with a local guest speaker discussing diet, nutrition, exercise, or mental health, followed by an open forum where women shared their challenges and successes. Ultimately, each would face the dreaded moment of truth—the public "weigh-in"—and if the scale's needle went in the wrong direction, the offender was made to stand in the "pig line." The group in the pig line was made to sing an embarrassingly silly jingle to the tune of the Yale "Whiffenpoof Song":

We are plump little pigs who ate too much, fat, fat, fat
We are stout little pigs who can't resist food, food, food
Pounds can be lost if you're really sincere
Pledge to TOPS for a year
Willpower helps us to be KOPS
TOPS, TOPS, TOPS

Then they paid a fine. By the end of the decade, there were 30,000 members. Today there are 170,000 men, women, and children in TOPS chapters worldwide. It is a not-for-profit organization with volunteer leaders, a $26 annual membership fee, and an association with the

73

TOPS Obesity and Metabolic Research Program at the Medical College of Wisconsin, established with a $4.5 million donation from TOPS. The weigh-in became private and confidential by the end of the 1950s, and Manz wrote a formal letter doing away with the "Pig Song" and other negative symbols in 1964. The TOPS Web site claims that in 2008, members lost more than 430 tons.

Various groups dedicated to weight loss began to form all over the country, some more effective and better executed than others. In 1951, a *New York Times* reporter enrolled in a typical ad hoc meeting on Manhattan's Lower East Side, where the slim nutritionist who was group leader turned dieting into a friendly competition among the exclusively female group. The session opened with a "weigh-in," followed by a discussion of food fads and positive strategies. Members shared everything from an uncontrollable passion for buttered English muffins to a story about a friend who, existing only on bananas and black coffee, had blacked out on the street the previous morning. In this predominantly Italian neighborhood, the leader gave an explanation of why a dinner made up of servings of meat, salad, vegetable, fruit, and milk was a healthier (if not tastier) choice than a big plate of pasta and meat sauce. Several members gave testament that they had never been able to lose weight by themselves, but now they were united and successful. Loosely formed "calorie clubs" where people socialized, learned how to prevent diabetes and obesity, and sometimes listened to music and danced gained in popularity. Group hypnosis, in which a few hundred overweight people at a time were put into a trance, was popular in San Jose, California. Hypnotherapist Herbert Mann, MD, claimed a success rate of 95 percent, explaining, "What we are really trying to do is to convert gross eaters into gourmets who would rather dine amid beautiful surroundings on dainty portions than gorge themselves on heavy servings of mashed potatoes and gravy. Men as well as women have responded to this therapy," he said.

THE FAT MAN'S CLUB

Obesity, which had formerly been considered a primarily female issue, officially became a problem for upper-middle-class men in 1952, when the American Medical Association (AMA) issued an alarming statement: "Overweight among American business executives is threatening destruction of the nation's productive capacity and free enterprise system." Antoinette Donnelly quickly shifted the responsibility to housewives. "STOP KILLING YOUR HUSBAND," she admonished in screamingly large type, telling readers that her anti-widowhood campaign was about to begin.

The Caterpillar Tractor Company in Peoria, Illinois, took swift action, blaming their executives' excess weight on noble causes like "worry and tensions, combined with enormous responsibilities to workers and stockholders." The company's medical director, Harold A. Vonachen, MD, believed that along with the stress, a lack of exercise and far too many highballs were also contributing to the excessive padding around the waistlines of Caterpillar's exclusively male top-management team. Bringing some of the new psychological jargon to the argument, he added that food was being used to compensate for these men's anxieties at work. He warned, "Industry might be able to afford losing its machines, but if it permits its executives to kill themselves from overeating, the country's know-how and productive genius which is preserving it as the last bulwark of democracy will be destroyed."

It is therefore not surprising that Vonachen organized a Fat Man's Club, where Lulu Hunt Peters was once again proved correct—it was a "disgrace" to be a member. The men ate meals together in the company dining room, carried around pocket calorie charts, and snatched food away from any members who seemed to be eating inappropriately. Vonachen reported that they were finding their "spiritual handles"—that is, they were now doing good and believing in God, something, apparently, they had been neglecting to do when they were eating themselves senseless.

Other large corporations, such as E. I. du Pont de Nemours and Company, where Alfred Pennington was testing his famous very-low-carb diets, began to develop their own weight-loss programs. Chase Manhattan Bank and Prudential Insurance offered low-calorie menus in their employee dining rooms. Since corporations were mainly concerned with people at or near the top of their food chains, an overweight manager was first to be placed in the crosshairs or, as the chairman of the committee on employment of the American Diabetes Association put it: "Start off with the executives!" Obesity was defined as a weight 20 percent above the Metropolitan Life Insurance Company recommendations for "ideal" weight. Remarks about "fat folks" were becoming increasingly prejudicial. "Fat workers are less efficient," it was said. "They are more accident prone," and "overweight workers are lower in productivity and higher in degenerative diseases." At the 1952 annual meeting of the AMA, Edward L. Bortz, MD, stated, "We're going to have to take off the kid gloves in dealing with people who are wallowing in their own grease."

LET'S WATCH OUR WEIGHT TOGETHER

William G. Wilson established Alcoholics Anonymous in 1940 based on his belief that a group of people with the same problem who are committed to supporting and respecting one another without judgment would heal more effectively together than alone. Overeaters Anonymous (OA), founded in 1960 by Rozanne S., a copywriter and the daughter of a dietitian, was similar to Alcoholics Anonymous. OA stressed that overweight and obesity were the results of addiction to food. Group support, individual sponsors, a progressive 12-step program, and a commitment to losing pounds slowly were the treatment. OA is still thriving as a nonprofit organization self-supported by member contributions.

In 1961, Jean Slutsky Nidetch, a 214-pound, 5-foot-7-inch, 38-year-old brunette from Little Neck, Long Island, went on a diet after running into a friend at the supermarket who exclaimed, "You look so marvelous. When are you due?" She had dieted many times before, trying everything from watermelon and black coffee to sunflower seeds, and always regained the weight she lost. This time, however, she was determined. This time would be different. She had an appointment at the New York City Department of Health's famous Obesity Clinic, run by Norman Jolliffe. Jolliffe combined a support group led by a well-credentialed nutritionist with education about long-term health maintenance.

Nidetch was given a goal weight of 142 pounds because she was told she had a "medium frame" (although she was positive it was really "large"). She pledged to follow the prescribed diet exactly as written. After looking it over, she realized that she already owned a copy. Not only was she addicted to food, she was also obsessed with dieting and cataloging hundreds of ways to reduce. She pasted diets into albums and stored the overflow in shoeboxes. She couldn't seem to be able to collect enough of them, as if just being aware of a variety of methods would empower her to lose weight.

Jolliffe's clinic was free, the stipulation being that if you didn't follow the rules, you would be asked to leave. Nidetch cheated. She lied. Finally, embarrassed and desperate, she called six "fat friends" and invited them over to her house to talk about what was happening. This informal group would become her contribution to Joliffe's program—talk therapy.

In her autobiography, *The Story of Weight Watchers,* Nidetch tells of convincing the original six to go on the diet with her, and how they then invited their friends, who invited theirs. Group support was the magic pill that Nidetch had been searching for. She lost 72 pounds, became a blonde, and began lecturing to large audiences while standing beside a photograph of the woman she had been. She urged all members to carry around photographs of their former bigger selves, saying, "I pray that I'll never forget where I came from." Eventually she began referring to herself as Jean Nidetch, FFH (Formally Fat Housewife), adding the self-deprecating initials after attending a by-invitation-only medical conference and being the only person in the room without initials after her name. Nidetch's Weight Watchers International was incorporated in 1963 at the encouragement of Albert Lippert, an overweight business-man who lost 40 pounds using her methods. The original board con-sisted of Lippert and his wife and Nidetch and her husband, Marty, who gave up his day job driving a bus along with 69 pounds. Five years later, there were 297 classes a week in New York City and 25 franchise opera-tions in 16 states, as well as others in London and Tel Aviv. Plans were in place for South America and South Africa. Nidetch estimated that half a million dieters had lost 10 million pounds with her help.

The H. J. Heinz Company bought Weight Watchers International in 1978 for $72 million. The sales growth was 15 percent a year; in 1986 the

New York Times referred to it as a "fat-reducing empire" with a magazine, cookbooks, and frozen foods. Today, at 4.7 percent of total sales, it has the largest market share of the American weight-loss industry. A current investors' report compiled by Oppenheimer Funds states, in the jargon typical of big-business investors' reports, "We continue to recommend [Weight Watchers International] for long-term investors looking to play the obesity theme."

AVERAGE BECOMES IDEAL AND DESIRABLE

In 1884, the Lithuanian parents of the future Louis I. Dublin, PhD, immigrated to America with their 2-year-old son. His father found work as a tailor on Manhattan's Lower East Side, and Louis, analytical and intelligent, was admitted to City College at the age of 14, where he majored in mathematics, and received a PhD in biology from Columbia University in 1904. In 1909, he went to work for the Metropolitan Life Insurance Company, where he stayed for more than 50 years. He became its statistician and communication strategist—the face of the company.

Dublin was a prolific researcher and writer, managing to easily maneuver back and forth between popular magazines and scientific journals on his key issues of public health and longevity. In 1933 he published, with coauthor Bessie Bunzel, *To Be, or Not to Be,* a 443-page statistical study of suicide indicating, among many other things, that men were more likely to end their lives than women, and black men more so than white. *The Psychoanalytic Review* called the work admirable, noting that Dublin seemed very aware that statistics only touched the surface of a problem so profoundly complex.

It is surprising that a man with such impressive credentials would develop Met Life's standardized weight charts using only data drawn from a predominantly white, male, East Coast population that included the very wealthy. These highly unscientific charts weren't only categorized by sex and height, they were also trifurcated by "frame size." Earlier charts termed the recommended weights "average," but by 1942 the median of this self-selecting group was referred to as "ideal." It was necessary to establish whether your build was small, medium, or large before you could determine if your weight was "ideal" or not, and although there was a way to do this, the method was both arbitrary and obscure.

To make a simple approximation of your frame size:

Extend your arm and bend the forearm upwards at a 90-degree angle. Keep the fingers straight and turn the inside of your wrist toward the body. Place the thumb and index finger of your other hand on the two prominent bones on either side of your elbow. Measure the space between your fingers against a ruler or a tape measure. (For the most accurate measurement, have your physician measure your elbow breadth with calipers.) Compare this measurement with the measurements shown below.

These tables list the elbow measurements for men and women of medium frame at various heights. Measurements lower than those listed indicate that you have a small frame while higher measurements indicate a large frame.

ELBOW MEASUREMENTS FOR MEDIUM FRAME

MEN		WOMEN	
HEIGHT (in 1-inch Heels)	ELBOW BREADTH (inches)	HEIGHT (in 1-inch Heels)	ELBOW BREADTH (inches)
5'2"–5'3"	$2\frac{1}{2}$"–$2\frac{7}{8}$"	4'10"–4'11"	$2\frac{1}{4}$"–$2\frac{1}{2}$"
5'4"–5'7"	$2\frac{5}{8}$"–$2\frac{7}{8}$"	5'0"–5'3"	$2\frac{1}{4}$"–$2\frac{1}{2}$"
5'8"–5'11"	$2\frac{3}{4}$"–3"	5'4"–5'7"	$2\frac{3}{8}$"–$2\frac{5}{8}$"
6'0"–6'3"	$2\frac{3}{4}$"–$3\frac{1}{8}$"	5'8"–5'11"	$2\frac{3}{8}$"–$2\frac{5}{8}$"
6'4"	$2\frac{7}{8}$"–$3\frac{1}{4}$"	6'0"	$2\frac{1}{2}$"–$2\frac{3}{4}$"

To complicate things even more, the definition of "ideal" would change every time new data was tabulated for publication. In 1942, the chart listed an adult 5-foot-4-inch woman's "ideal" weight as being between 116 and 142 pounds when "ordinarily dressed, with shoes." In 1959, the "desirable" weight for a woman of the same height was between 108 and 138 pounds "in indoor clothing, with shoes." (By 1983, the chart had been renamed, simply, a "weight chart" and recommended that the

5-foot-4-inch woman weigh 114 to 151 pounds wearing "indoor clothing weighing 3 pounds and shoes with 1" heels.") Like Jean Nidetch, most people just considered themselves "big-boned" (and overdressed) and were satisfied as long as they fit into any of the categories listed for their height.

Dublin's charts set the standard for body weight. Norman Jolliffe was one of many physicians who used them with his patients. The charts were attached to public scales and printed many times over in books and magazines—it would have been difficult not to know your average, ideal, desirable weight. Since Metropolitan Life believed that slim policyholders represented fat profits, they aimed to create a world where everyone was "ideal."

Although others had said it before, it was Dublin who made it stick. "Obesity is America's number one health problem!" he proclaimed in 1951, and he used the phrase again as the title of an article in *Today's Health* magazine the following year. A public relations expert and scientist, Dublin created a slogan with staying power. He used the Met Life Insurance statistics to link obesity to a shortened life span. While that may have been true, policyholders were weighed only when they bought insurance—nothing was known about their lifestyles after that until their heirs presented their death certificates. Exercise, diet, smoking, alcohol consumption, travel, occupation, emotional well-being, and genetic predispositions weren't taken into consideration by Dublin in his life-expectancy projections. It seems odd, given that as a student, he had done a good deal of research in the area of insect chromosomes and genetics, as well as work that had, at one point, been praised for its acute sensitivity to statistics. It is possible that Dublin so deeply believed that there was a growing problem of obesity that he overlooked adherence to some of his scientific methods. It is also feasible that his employer's interests might have factored into his recommendations.

In 1951, Dublin's latest statistics were based on a long-range study of more than 50,000 men and women who were insured as "sub-standards," which meant that they carried policies that cost more because they were categorized as obese. He and a colleague initially presented their results at the afternoon closing session of the 60th annual meeting of the Association of Life Insurance Medical Directors of America in New York City, an event widely covered by the press. They reported that there was a strong correlation between obesity and early death from diabetes and degenerative diseases of the kidneys, liver, and heart. The death rate for obese men from 20 to 29 years old, at 214 percent above normal, was of particular significance, as was the evidence that an overweight woman was more likely to die in childbirth. The rates of mortality among the overweight increased in direct proportion to the degree of overweight, and encouragingly, those who lost weight lived longer than those who did not. (Dublin determined this by comparing mortality on policies issued as substandard with those initially issued as substandard but later reissued as standard when their holders requested they be reevaluated due to weight loss. However, these subjects were never weighed a third time, and nothing else was known about them until they died.) Standard and substandard groups showed no difference in mortality rates from cancer, and death from tuberculosis was significantly *lower* among the overweight population. These were interesting and, at the time, underplayed statistical findings, because they didn't prove his point. However, aggregate mortality for the substandard group was 50 percent higher than for the standards between the ages of 20 and 64, and that was the takeaway. "Excess weight carries very definite penalties in terms of health and longevity," Dublin concluded. This strengthened his company's platform that the elimination of many infectious diseases along with the easy availability of plentiful food was causing a new epidemic: the obesity epidemic.

WEIGHT-LOSS NATION

Metropolitan Life suggested a solution for America's fat problem: Every American should lose 20 pounds, for a combined national weight loss of more than half a billion pounds. Met Life stated that the country's high standard of living resulted in the highest obesity rates in the world. They were given the full support of the US Public Health Service and the AMA, both of whom accepted Dublin's conclusions. Both organizations agreed that the only way to reduce was to eat less. Pills and starvation diets didn't work. But group support was highly recommended because, as Met

Life's vice president in charge of health and welfare, D. B. Armstrong, MD, put it, "It makes it a lot easier when one waistline watcher can boast of his achievements to another, or find out how a fellow sufferer got through that first awful week." *Cheers for Chubby*, an 8-minute animated color film created and distributed by the insurance company, was distributed to movie theaters throughout the country to offer additional encouragement, and a new company pamphlet, *Overweight and Underweight*, was available upon request, free of charge, to help struggling people on either side of the balancing scale. Met Life even rolled out a new slogan: "The longer the belt line, the shorter the life line."

Nutritionists and physicians were alarmed. It was estimated that 10 percent of people in large cities were now overweight, and it was "common knowledge" that the plague of obesity was the number one health problem in America. The connection between diabetes, heart disease, and obesity appeared irrefutable. The *Washington Post* proclaimed obesity "a national health menace" and, in 1951, estimated that 25 to 30 percent of American adults were as much as 20 pounds overweight; these numbers now seem prescient, but quaint. The country, at least the white middle class, and especially white middle-class women, seemed ready to accept the edict that they needed to lose a few pounds.

THE GOLDEN AGE OF CHAINS

A victorious, prosperous, hungry, and in actuality only mildly weight-challenged America was poised to undergo a revolution in its approach to mealtime. Never a country with particularly high culinary ambitions and always quick to embrace science and technology to the detriment of taste, much American fare remained relatively uninspired. There were exceptions, of course, including some excellent home cooks and expensive big-city restaurants, but overall this lackluster cuisine was the perfect foundation for two significant changes—fast food and chemicals. After Harvey Wiley revealed the dangers of preservatives, American food might have been bland, but it was also relatively unadulterated for decades. When people today complain that chicken, strawberries, or tomatoes just don't taste the way they used to, you can bet they either grew up on farms or are old enough to remember the taste of the pre-factory food of the 1940s.

Food could be purchased and consumed quickly at luncheonette counters and drive-ins throughout the country before fast food outlets became ubiquitous, but that food was cooked to order, sometimes with expertise and care, sometimes not. In 1948, brothers Richard and Maurice McDonald decided to convert their traditional carhop-style 1940 San Bernardino, California, drive-in—which had an extensive and unwieldy menu—to a restaurant that served only a very limited selection of fresh and deliciously prepared bestsellers—hamburgers (no more meat rationing!), milkshakes, and french fries kept hot and ready to go under their innovative infrared heat lamps. They were so successful that by 1952 they had opened six more outlets. Two years later they had eight, and Ray Kroc, a 52-year-old Multimixer milkshake machine salesman curious to know how just one of those restaurants could need eight mixers, flew to the West Coast and had the idea that changed the American landscape and made him one of the wealthiest men in the world. He requested and received the rights to open a franchise operation, and in 1955 Kroc opened his first McDonald's in Des Plaines, Illinois, with a limited menu similar to the McDonalds' restaurant that included hamburgers (15 cents), cheeseburgers (19 cents), french fries (10 cents), soft drinks (10 cents or 15 cents), vanilla and chocolate shakes (20 cents), and coffee (10 cents). By 1960, his chain was grossing $56 million a year; in 1961 he paid the McDonald brothers $2.7 million for everything, including their name. In 2007, it was reported to be a $22.8 billion company, making it by far the largest fast food corporation in the world.

The decade of the 1950s is accurately referred to as the golden age of American food chains. An abbreviated time line of foundings reads as follows: Dunkin' Donuts, 1950; Taco Bell, 1952; Burger King, 1954; Ray Kroc's McDonald's, 1955; Kentucky Fried Chicken, 1955; Pizza Hut, 1958; International House of Pancakes, 1958; and Domino's Pizza, 1960. New highways, affordable automobiles, mass-produced suburbs, the baby boom, women remaining in or returning to the workforce, dual-income families, and the stirrings of another feminist movement—all of these things came together at the right time, enabling the fast food industry to flourish. It never could have grown so rapidly and successfully, however, if it hadn't also coincided with the golden age of American food chemistry. From 1949 to 1959, chemists developed more than 400 new additives that allowed food to travel thousands of miles and remain "fresh," extending its shelf life from a few days to months. Growth hormones administered to bovines made dairy cows lactate longer and steers grow bigger faster and on less feed. Antibiotics became staples of livestock production, allowing more than 40,000 chickens to be crowded into stifling, windowless coops that once held only a fraction of that number and thousands of cattle to be crammed into grassless feedlots on land that had once supported just a few herds. The drugs made them disease resistant, an imperative in the filthy, close quarters. Food animals were no longer treated as living creatures capable of feeling pleasure, discomfort, and pain. They were transformed into inorganic manufactured parts to be wrapped in cellophane and Styrofoam and stacked on supermarket shelves. Without ever having had a life even remotely worth living, they now appeared never to have lived at all.

LOTS OF FOOD, GLORIOUS FOOD

Such an extreme surplus of beef and milk was available that the government began touting the benefits of beef stew in marketing campaigns. Eisenhower was having beef stew luncheons, and Dairy Month—June— was created to deal with the dairy surplus. There was overproduction of potatoes, carrots, and onions as well—ingredients for the stew. Food had always been inexpensive in America compared with the rest of the world, and now it was downright cheap. It was also less flavorful; therefore the development of chemical flavoring agents became important.

This radical shift from whole to highly processed foods was propelled by the Eisenhower administration when he came into office in 1953. Although the FDA, suspicious about potential carcinogens, was requesting that manufacturers conduct more research on all of the additives and enhancers, the new president (who had a farm in Gettysburg, Pennsylvania, and enjoyed the fresh vegetables grown there) didn't believe the government should interfere with private industry. He didn't want to quash American optimism or the global perception of the United States as the

84

richest, best-fed country in the world. To drive this point home, soon after his inauguration he attended a luncheon at the USDA research facilities in Beltsville, Maryland, to celebrate some of the new "miracle" foods. The feast included powdered orange juice, whey cheese spread, dehydrofrozen (partially dehydrated and then frozen) peas, and beef and pork laced with hormones and antibiotics. Secretary of agriculture Ezra Taft Benson, attending a luncheon for journalists, predicted that they could all look forward to some "amazing advances." Powdered fruit concentrates would be joined by frozen and powdered milk, all poultry would be either canned or frozen, and eggs would be indefinitely "fresh." Innovation would save the American diet. The days of Grandma needing to visit the market for fresh food each day and slaving over a hot stove to prepare it were, mercifully, over.

Despite the national weight-loss campaigns under way at the time, the 1950s presented the perfect circumstances for fattening up. The middle class's move to the suburbs resulted in their driving more and walking less; working mothers and dual-income families gladly relied on all of the new fast food restaurants, TV dinners, and other frozen convenience meals; televisions kept people, especially children, indoors and inactive; and the hour devoted to physical education was disappearing from many public schools. In addition to exercising less, people were eating more of the cheap, readily available surplus food. In 1952, the Bureau of Agricultural Economics reported an increase in per capita food consumption of 12 percent over the 1935 to 1939 time period. There may have been a lot of talk about the necessity to lose weight in the 1930s, but collectively, Americans kept their weight stable during the Great Depression, the Great War, and World War II. But now food had never been so plentiful and cheap, and people were taking advantage of the bounty.

The belts were getting longer, and there were new ideas about what you could do about it. You could, for example, try Dr. Jonas's methylcellulose tablets. He had finally gotten them to market under the name Wafex ("No Calorie Counting!" "No Diets!" "No Exercises!"). This $3-a-month "food adjunct" was advertised as being so filling that just one 5-calorie wafer had the "hunger-satisfying" capability of five slices of white bread, four eggs, and a pound of boiled potatoes. Exercising was said to be useless, since it was purported to be scientific fact that a person would have to walk at least 30 miles to lose a pound. The converse, that walking 1 mile a day for 30 days would keep a pound away, was for the moment conveniently ignored. *Time* magazine quoted a physician at an AMA meeting in Chicago as stating that to lose a pound, you would have to climb the Washington Monument 48 times or do 2,400 pushups. What was the point?

WHERE DIET IS A FOUR-LETTER WORD

When Lawrence L. Mack left the US Navy at the end of World War II, he developed the brilliant but worthless theory of "passive exercise." His first four Slenderella International reducing salons opened for business in 1950 in New York City, charging $2 per session. By 1954 he owned 91 salons, and by 1956 there were 110. Mack was committing seven-figure sums to radio, television, and print ads. It was a perfect scheme, because, like Wafex, no diet or exercise was required (and unlike Wafex, you could still enjoy a good meal). The salons catered to a female clientele (according to the *New York Times*, the narrow silhouette of the new and trendy sheath dress was sending women there by the thousands), and their ads promised "no disrobing, dull, exhausting exercise, or starvation diets."

The word "diet" was not allowed utterance at Slenderalla studios, and the first visit was free. The client was measured and then directed to her small cubicle. Once there, she was told to lie down on a vibrating table with the assurance that all of the shaking would "firm and mold." After the "treatment," she received her menu plans, a box of Slenderella vitamin mints, and direction on how many times she would need to return to achieve her goal weight. By 1959, there were 150 salons in the United States, Canada, and Europe, grossing more than $25 million annually. The chain closed that year, after Mack's assets were frozen and liens were put on his business due to tax fraud—Mack owed the IRS more than $1 million.

In some cities, Slenderella salons had competition. Washington, DC, ladies could switch to the rival Stauffer System salons, where a sign on the wall read: "Horses or women / It doesn't matter / A sway in the back / Makes them all look fatter." The Stauffer System focused on posture-improvement classes, followed by a vibrating treatment in a small, curtained cubicle where soft music relaxed the passive exerciser. It was a popular diversion. There was no diet, but a "sensible eating" plan was suggested and "appetite appeasing" wafers were available to snack on.

The RelaxAcizor was a portable electric machine for people who wanted the passive exercise experience at home. After applying a "special" cream, the user attached contact pads and electrodes to his or her fat-challenged body parts. Electric charges then repeatedly contracted the muscles. That was all there was to the "exercise" part of the procedure; the manufacturer claimed the pounds would effortlessly disappear. It was predicted that $1 billion worth of home massage units, as they were called, would be sold by the end of the decade. The FDA prohibited the sale of the RelaxAcizor beginning in 1970 and also demanded that all existing machines be destroyed because they could cause heart arrhythmias and miscarriages and worsen epilepsy, ulcers, and hernias. More than 400,000 had been sold. The Hip Shaker, a ridiculous contraption that encircled the hips and vibrated while the dieter stood still, replaced it.

8

"HOW DO I LOSE WEIGHT *FAST?*"

IN 1901, THE INFANT GRANDSON OF JOHN D. ROCKEFELLER—AMERICA'S FIRST BILLIONAIRE—became ill with scarlet fever. Even Rockefeller's unlimited wealth and medical contacts couldn't save the life of a baby who had contracted a deadly infectious disease at a time before there was any known cure. This tragedy inspired Rockefeller to fast-track a vision he had held on to for years: He would build and finance a facility modeled on France's Pasteur Institute. This research laboratory, to be the first of its kind in America, would be devoted solely to discovering the underlying causes of the deadliest diseases, such as scarlet fever, diphtheria, and typhoid fever. In 1903, he paid $700,000 to purchase the largest piece of unimproved property in New York City available south of Harlem. It had once been the elegant Schermerhorn Farm on York Avenue between 64th and 67th streets, and it was situated high atop a bluff that sloped down to the East River. Because city authorities were willing to erase any projected street extensions, the beautiful property could remain contiguous, and construction began immediately on magnificent buildings to house scientists, technicians, and laboratory animals. In 1910, the first hospital in America devoted exclusively to clinical research was opened on the property as well.

At the time, it was theorized that milk might contain bacteria that contributed to childhood diseases, and so the Rockefeller Institute sent teams of researchers to investigate the city's milk supply. Reports were filed stating that although some farms followed sanitary practices, others were filthy. Cows were milked by workers with dirty hands; the fresh milk flowed into unwashed pails and was shipped without ice from upstate New York to the lower reaches of Manhattan in the summer heat. Samples of grocery store milk showed dangerously high levels of bacteria. This project initiated regulatory changes to methods of milk processing and distribution that proved important to the welfare of the city. Rockefeller's institute attracted top scientific talent, and it thrived.

By midcentury, the discovery of antibiotics had greatly reduced mortality rates for infectious diseases. With one public health risk attended to, the focus shifted to cardiovascular diseases. And at the institute, Vincent P. Dole, MD, was specifically concerned with metabolic disorders. As evidence linking heart disease to elevated blood cholesterol levels and obesity mounted, a series of weight-loss experiments were conducted at the elite institute, which, in 1956, had transitioned into a graduate university granting a combined degree of doctor of medical science and doctor of philosophy.

Dole's research suggested that obesity was a symptom of an underlying metabolic disorder that might be improved with a low-protein, calorically *un*restricted diet. This resulted in two promising new weight-loss strategies that Dole warned should be undertaken only within the confines of a tightly controlled scientific environment. Nevertheless, rumors about these amazing new diets began to spread. One was a liquid diet that would soon be referred to as the Fabulous Formula or the Crash Diet in women's magazines, while the other, which permitted solid food, was known simply as the Rockefeller Diet. The solid diet was low in protein, but it didn't eliminate sugar or fat, which added to its appeal. The liquid diet, a mixture of corn oil, dextrose, evaporated milk, and water, was a fair approximation of human breast milk.

STARVED AND STUFFED

While these new weight-loss methods were being tested, an obese, legally blind man in his forties applied for an entry-level administrative position at the beautiful Rockefeller facility on the Upper East Side of Manhattan.

Baron Roy Andries de Groot was the Oxford-educated son of a French noblewoman, the husband of the successful British actress Katherine Hynes, and a sophisticated journalist and epicure, making him an unusual candidate for what was essentially a clerical job. Still, he was hired, in that very different time, after explaining that he was a writer planning a book set in a hospital and was in need of background information. Actually, de Groot had heard from a Canadian doctor friend that the institute was experimenting with new, fail-proof methods of weight loss, and he wanted not only to write about what they were doing, but also to volunteer as a subject.

He loved food with the kind of passion that made him the founder and first president of the International Gourmet Society, as well as eventually an outstanding food writer and cookbook author. He wasn't always a heavy man; the extra pounds were added after a German air raid on Britain during World War II injured him so grievously that he was forced to lie sandbagged in bed for several months. He also later lost his eyesight due to the incident. Since he was devoted to cooking and eating well, family members read the writings of legendary French chef and culinary writer Auguste Escoffier aloud to him on a daily basis as diversion. His health improved, as did his eyesight initially, but only temporarily—he eventually became legally blind and would frequently be seen shopping for food in Greenwich Village accompanied by his beloved Alsatian guide dog. He obsessively cooked for his wife and two young daughters. There weren't enough meals in a day, or courses in a meal, and he just kept cooking, and eating, and gaining more weight.

At the time of his job application at the institute, he weighed 281 pounds. His young doctor friend had told him that some people, unlike most, didn't know when to stop eating, and that some could lose weight and keep it off while others couldn't, but no one could yet explain why. However, scientists at the Rockefeller Institute were experimenting with a way to alter metabolism. This was a method whereby you "cut way down on certain foods and gorge on all the others." This was a whole new way of thinking about food—"the stuffing is fun and the starving goes unnoticed." This was revolutionary.

De Groot managed to become a test subject, and he lost 45 pounds in 3 months. In June 1956, his book about the experience was published: *How I Reduced with the New Rockefeller Diet: Part 1. The Rockefeller Diet. Part 2. The Diet for Gourmets*. At once autobiography, history, cookbook, and conveyor of the coveted solid-food version of the diet, this is probably the most enjoyable and erudite book ever written on how to lose weight, although admittedly the literary diet-book genre doesn't see a lot of competition.

For the first month, de Groot ate only carefully controlled portions of fruit juices, soups, vegetables, and salads, with a few slices of bread, a little bit of protein, and some potatoes and pasta—but all the butter, oil, and jam he wanted. This made his daily allotment of bread quite delicious, served alongside a gigantic salad tossed with lovely, freshly made vinaigrette. This was a reasonable plan, especially for someone who knew his way around salad dressings and jam. Everything he ate had to be written down exactly as consumed. After 4 weeks, he could enjoy a glass or two of wine daily. The Rockefeller Diet was a plant-based, low-calorie, low-protein diet, and it would be difficult not to lose weight if followed correctly. It was also a pleasant way of eating for life—a blueprint for Michael Pollan's well-put directive to "eat food. Not too much. Mostly plants," and similar to the one recommended by Russell Chittenden at Yale University in 1910.

De Groot wrote in his best-selling book that the plan had "civilized my eating," noting that MIT biochemistry professor Robert Harris, PhD, said that although the natural instinct of all creatures is to eat in a healthy manner, those instincts had been crushed in America. "It is not true that the people of the U.S. are the best fed people in the world. Americans seem to be befuddled by the enormous variety of processed foods available from the U.S. food industry," wrote de Groot.

FAST AND EASY:
THE AMERICAN WAY OF DIETING

Robert Waithman, a British journalist who reported on American politics and culture for the *New York Times,* wrote in a story published in that newspaper that eating in America has become a "joyless" activity.

With 60 percent of the nation's women and 20 percent of its men on diets, he was probably right. Eat a little bit less of what you like, he suggested, and even if that happens to be bread and cheese, you'll do just fine. He described conversations he would have with American friends who had just returned from Italy or France raving about how they had the *best* beef, tomatoes, or vegetables of their lives in Europe. He asked them: "Isn't it just possible the food wasn't processed, tenderized, frozen or what have you?"

De Groot, enthralled with his own success on the Rockefeller Diet (his book had not yet been published), responded with an angry letter to the editor. Waithman may not realize it, he wrote, but appreciation for fine food was on the rise in America. De Groot suggested that many of the 44 million people Waithman said were "dieting" had simply learned the basics of sound nutrition and were consuming appropriate amounts of delicious, *unprocessed* steaks, chickens, salmon, fruits, vegetables, and wine; already limiting their intake of bread and cheese; and eliminating dessert completely, thank you very much. The letter was signed "Roy de Groot, President, International Gourmet Society."

For de Groot and his society pals, this may well have been true. But for the most part, Waithman, the foreign observer, had gotten it right. Americans *were* searching for the perfect diet, and they wanted one even simpler than de Groot's short list of easily available, unprocessed foods. They demanded fail-safe, instant results, no matter how punishing or tortuous the regimen. The prize was in the losing, not in the maintaining. They wanted the Fabulous Formula!

To that end, in August 1956, the *other* famous Rockefeller Institute diet was added to de Groot's book, and a revised edition containing the Formula diet was published.

LIQUID ASSETS

That Fabulous Formula became readily available to consumers after Mead Johnson and Company more or less replicated the Rockefeller Institute recipe and sold it first in powdered form as Enfamil, an infant formula with the composition of human breast milk, and then as Sustagen, a meal replacement for invalids unable to eat solid food. In 1959, in a stroke of marketing genius, executives realized that the drink was often consumed by neither infants nor invalids, but by adults trying to lose weight. In fact, that was happening more than ever since the new Metropolitan Life Insurance Company weight charts had come out. Chemists increased the formula's protein content and transformed it into a "metered-calorie product" called Metrecal. In less than a year a whole new market was born. The *New York Times* called it the latest rage for "those who need to reduce or think they do," adding that discussions of favorite flavors (the choices were chocolate, vanilla, and butterscotch) were overheard at parties all over town.

Mead Johnson was known as an ethical company, meaning the majority of its products were available by prescription only. Initial advertisements for Metrecal appeared only in the pages of the *Journal of the American Medical Association*. When Mead Johnson broadened the campaign, its ads recommended consulting with a physician and presented a somber and scientific page of information, lending the over-the-counter Metrecal the illusion of being an FDA-approved prescription.

Losing weight the Metrecal way was foolproof, especially since within the first year it became available premixed in serving-size cans that required no refrigeration. All you had to do was drink four glasses of the flavored beverage a day. This would supply about 900 daily calories, so it wasn't surprising when a study conducted at the Good Samaritan Hospital in Phoenix showed that 97 out of 100 people who followed the four-glasses-a-day plan lost an average of $\frac{1}{2}$ pound daily. (What about the 3 percent who didn't lose weight even when starved? The question was never raised.)

There had never been a diet craze like this one, according to *Time* magazine. You were practically guaranteed to lose $3\frac{1}{2}$ pounds a week, and you didn't have to shop or cook! Mead Johnson's earnings for the first half of 1960 were pushed to record levels, and its net profits almost doubled.

By 1961, there were more than 100 meal replacement products on the market; by 1963, there were more than 700. Sears, Roebuck and Company called it Bal-Cal; Quaker Oats named it Quota; and Pet Milk introduced Sego, although Metrecal by any other name was still baby formula mixed with water and a poor excuse for food. Nevertheless, liquid meals began appearing on restaurant menus across America. Businessmen at Denver's exclusive Twenty-Six Club ordered it, and Chicago's Union League Club reported that it served 100 glasses a week at 65 cents each. President John F. Kennedy's staff could choose from two flavors in their private White House lunchroom. The king of Greece had cases shipped in. So did the royal families of Saudi Arabia. Stanley Marcus, founder of the specialty store Neiman-Marcus, said that he liked to mix Metrecal with tomato paste, cucumbers, ground-up peppers, tomatoes, and curry powder to make "a kind of Spanish gazpacho soup." Indeed, a lot of users needed to mix it with something. Trader Vic's, a trendy restaurant chain, offered this 325-calorie, $1.50 lunch: 1½ ounces of rum mixed with nutmeg, and Metrecal. What a delicious combination of infantilism and grown-up decadence, all in a tall and frosty glass.

DIET FOOD FIGHT

Just when Metrecal seemed to have established a firm grip on the liquid diet market, along came Sego with a wide variety of flavors, including orange, banana, chocolate malt, and pineapple. Sego also offered pudding and soup. Metrecal countered with prepared dinners and cookies, correctly assuming that dieters might want solid food and dessert now and then, but still, Metrecal's sales continued to deteriorate. In the 1970s, Pillsbury introduced Figurines diet candy bars and temporarily had the competition for lunch. Two Figurines contained 550 calories and were advertised as a balanced meal. Pillsbury's research had indicated that a product that was able to satisfy a dieter's craving for sweets could corner the whole diet market. The company's research also indicated that a lot of people seemed to enjoy the sensation of chewing.

The Metrecal brand was discontinued by Mead Johnson in the early 1980s, when Carnation Slender and then the brilliantly named Slim-Fast captured the market with aggressive promotion and pricing. Liquid diets and accessory products like meal replacement bars and cookies continue to thrive today in spite of the fact that they do nothing to change a dieter's long-term eating habits and are often just "nonfattening" snacks. In 2000,

Unilever paid $2.3 billion to acquire Slim-Fast Foods. It currently owns the third-largest share of the weight-loss market.

HAVING YOUR CAKE AND EATING IT, TOO

The liquid diets and meal replacement products that became pervasive at midcentury ultimately gave rise to a gigantic new segment of the food industry. There was a hunger for anything that had only a few calories and still tasted, more or less, like food.

Tillie Lewis, a Brooklyn-born entrepreneur who moved to California to prove that the tasty Italian pomodoro tomato could be grown domestically, was one of the first to figure this out. An early believer in day care centers, incentive plans, and easy transportation for workers who lived far from her factory, she was known to treat employees so well that the American Federation of Labor made an exception and didn't call workers to the picket line at Lewis's company during the 1940 California statewide cannery strike. In 1951, the Associated Press named her businesswoman of the year. Innovative and expansive, in 1953 she gambled that America was about to go on a nationwide diet. Tasti-Diet, her sugar- and salt-free line of canned fruits, puddings, jellies, and salad dressings, standardized artificially sweetened foods and made them widely available for the first time.

By 1957, at the 15th annual Newspaper Food Editors Conference, it was reported that almost 100 percent of newly opened supermarkets were stocking diet foods. The category had increased 500 percent in 5 years and was outselling baby food during the baby boom. There were low-calorie/low-sodium prepared fruits, vegetables, soups, cereals, dinner entrees like beef stew and chicken fricassee, cookies, salad dressings, candies, cake mixes, and chewing gums. As counterpoints to diet foods, the other trendy new products introduced at the conference were high-calorie and highly profitable "convenience meats" presented by the meat-packing giants Armour (frozen breaded veal drumsticks and a 4-ounce jar of dried beef with an attached foil cup holding concentrated white sauce) and Swift (chopped ham formed into sticks that were packed into a 14-ounce tin and named Ham Quick). The country was eating "lite"

95

foods, to be sure, but often in addition to, and not to substitute for, products like Ham Quick.

LET'S DRINK TO OUR HEALTH AND WEALTH

Hyman Kirsch, a Russian immigrant living in Brooklyn, was a successful manufacturer of ginger ale when he became vice president of the Jewish Sanitarium and Hospital for Chronic Diseases. In his new post he realized that the large number of diabetics wanted to drink soda, but weren't able to on their sugar-free diets. He and his son Morris worked with a research chemist to test various sugar substitutes. They rejected saccharin as tasting too metallic, but didn't mind the taste of calcium cyclamate at all, which was the artificial sweetener they ended up using in their new recipe. In 1952, No-Cal, the first diet soda, was born.

Soon available in six different flavors at less than 2 calories a glass, it became a regional East Coast success, selling 3 million cases in its first year on sale. A survey conducted by Grey Advertising in New York revealed that at least half of the buyers were not diabetic, just calorie conscious, and the company shifted its marketing efforts in that direction. Diet-Rite Cola, made by Royal Crown, a Midwest competitor, was introduced in 1958 and successfully marketed nationwide in 1962. At less than 3 calories a bottle, it looked and tasted like a cola drink. The following year, the Coca-Cola Company and the Pepsi-Cola Company introduced low-calorie soft drinks.

Sometimes it is the independent visionary, unhindered by a corporate culture of decision-making-by-committee and bureaucratic entanglements, who develops the most innovative new products. Brooklyn entrepreneur Benjamin Eisenstadt, for example, brought Sweet'N Low to market in 1957, as opposed to a pharmaceutical company or sugar refinery. And it was Hyman Kirsch who recognized the burgeoning trend of low-calorie soft drinks—and quickly capitalized on it—as industry giants Coke and Pepsi watched. Coke and Pepsi were reluctant to tinker with their hugely successful formulas. In their view, marketing diet cola might suggest that something was wrong with "the real thing." Top executives might even have thought it inconceivable that customers would want anything but the original version.

But just in case they did, the new drinks had better not compete with the old.

And so arrived Tab, the Coca-Cola Company's entry in the market, with the slogan "How can just one calorie taste so good?" In August 1963, a Coca-Cola spokesperson said its sales were "almost unbelievable," and that a huge ad campaign was planned for the following year. Pepsi's candidate, Patio Diet Cola, was also a success, and even more so after the name was changed to Diet Pepsi. In 1965, Coke had another successful introduction with its "adult" drink, Fresca, but the company refused to dilute the name Coke until 1982, when "the most significant new product introduction in the history of the company," diet (with a little d) Coke appeared "just for the taste of it." The problem, according to Marty Solow, the Brooklyn-born advertising man whose agency, Solow/Wexton, had acquired the No-Cal account from Grey, was that as Americans became more affluent, they became more married to the foods they loved. His theory, which he stated in Damon Runyon–like cadence, was "Their unconscious can be jolted, stimulated, by the suggestion that maybe if they drank this nice soda, they would eat with impunity the foods they should not be eating. This would give them a certain freedom." In other words, drink No-Cal *with* your dessert. His new print campaign consisted of full-page ads in *Life* and the *New York Times Magazine* showing a frosty glass of No-Cal surrounded by cake, cream pie, pudding topped with mounds of whipped cream, and other irresistible desserts. His slogan asks, "What's No-Cal doing with that rich crowd?" The campaign, although clever, was ultimately unsuccessful. With an advertising budget too small to include television, No-Cal was unable to compete. However, it reinforced the illogical concept that if you drank diet soda or, by extension, artificially sweetened your coffee or ate diet food products, you were doing something positive for your waistline no matter what else you ate. Meanwhile, newly named "health nuts" at Los Angeles juice bars were ordering pink, "high-protein" beverages made from dried eggs, powdered milk, and cherry-flavored No-Cal. An 8-ounce glass cost 59 cents.

Other companies tried to capture small pieces of the market with unusual, and also generally unsuccessful, offerings. Dr. Pepper, America's first soft drink company, created Pommac, an odd beverage that was supposed to taste like diet cognac. The IRS's closing of the Slenderella reducing salons (which in turn bankrupted Slenderella "magic skin" girdles, hosiery, and artificially sweetened foods) left the name up for grabs, and Walter S. Mack, formerly the president of the Pepsi-Cola Company and the current owner of C&C Cola, claimed it for his own with the short-lived "vitamin 'C' enriched" 1-calorie Slenderella, a "new diet high-carbonated soft drink."

Interestingly, as the diet soda market expanded, so did the nation's waistlines. Between 1965 and 2002, our per capita caloric intake from beverages doubled from 200 to 400 per day, with most of the increase coming from soda and fruit juice.

SWEETLY ARTIFICIAL

"Under the name of saccharin, a substance has recently attracted notice, both in Europe and America, that seems destined to play no small role commercially" began an article in the June 1886 *American Journal of Pharmacy*. This amazing "white, crystalline substance" derived from coal tar had a "peculiar quality of sweetness" and was about to become the first food coveted for having no nutritional value whatsoever. Many chemical "preservatives" had been added to foods, often illegally, but saccharin would become an ingredient in its own right. "Not a carbohydrate but a nitrogenous body" was how the journal put it, adding that the name was deceptive, since *saccharum* was the Latin word for "sugar." Still, it was stated, it might be a potentially useful sugar substitute for both diabetics and the obese.

By 1890, it was being prescribed for both, and used as a preservative too. In 1908, Harvey Washington Wiley, head of the FDA, considered it a dangerous (and deceptive) substance. In his autobiography, Wiley recalls an unfortunate experience he had in presenting his case to President Theodore Roosevelt, Secretary of Agriculture James Wilson, and several industry lobbyists: "President Roosevelt turned upon me, purple with anger, and with clenched fists, hissing through his teeth, said: 'You say saccharin is injurious to health? Why, Doctor Rixey gives it to me every day. Anybody who says saccharin is injurious to health is an idiot.'" Roosevelt believed so strongly in the substance (or its lobbyists) that he appointed a separate national committee of scientists to investigate saccharin; in 1910, they pronounced it safe in moderation.

Saccharin, however, was of limited usefulness. Some thought it had an unpleasant aftertaste, and it was inappropriate for cooking or baking because it decomposed at high heat. Still, it had no competition until, in 1950, Abbott Laboratories introduced Sucaryl, which had been first identified as an artificial sweetener in 1937 when a cigarette-smoking chemist noticed that his cigarettes tasted like sugar when he was experimenting with cyclamate. Sucaryl became available in tiny tablets, like saccharin, and also as a liquid, and as such began to frequently appear in diet recipes.

However, both products still had limitations. Neither, for example, could be satisfactorily sprinkled on a weight watcher's morning grapefruit. In 1957, Ben Eisenstadt, who owned Cumberland Packing, a company that packaged sugar and other condiments into sanitary individual packets for restaurant table service, created the no-calorie granulated sugar substitute Sweet'N Low, a combination of saccharin, cyclamate, and lactose. (When the FDA banned cyclamate as a carcinogen in 1969, Eisenstadt immediately switched to his not yet marketed formula for an all-saccharin, lactose-free, kosher Sweet'N Low, which became the market leader for years. In 1977, the FDA made manufacturers put a warning label on products containing saccharin.)

Other calorie-free sweeteners were developed, like aspartame (NutraSweet and Equal) and sucralose (Splenda). The latest is stevia.

In 1987, the *New York Times* published a history of sugar substitutes, including a long list of all of the cancer and other health scares that have accompanied them. Whether or not artificial sweeteners are dangerous is still being researched, and to date they seem to be what the FDA refers to as GRAS (generally recognized as safe).

Foods sweetened with any of them are a significant market, but not nearly as large as one would think. Currently, only about 15 percent of Americans consume any artificially sweetened products on a regular basis, and that includes soda.

9

PURE, WHITE, AND DEADLY

IN 1954, THE SUGAR INDUSTRY HIRED THE LEO BURNETT ADVERTISING AGENCY IN Chicago to begin a $1.8 million "educational" campaign aimed at teaching Americans the rightful place of sugar in a balanced diet. A year earlier, the American Sugar Refining Company, the huge conglomerate that sold sugar under the brand name Domino, hired a different agency, Ted Bates and Company, to combat the idea that sugar is fattening. The agency had conducted a survey and found that most women weren't aware of the caloric content of their food, so Bates was confident that their campaign would be successful. The idea was to associate sugar with foods perceived as nonfattening. For example, 3 teaspoons of sugar would be shown next to half a grapefruit to communicate that the sugar had slightly fewer calories. The claim was accurate, but misleading. The grapefruit half was the caloric equivalent of about 3 teaspoons of sugar—60 calories—but it also contained more than the minimum daily requirement of vitamin C, plus vitamin A, calcium, other nutrients, and fiber. The sugar contained 18 "empty" calories per teaspoon—no vitamins, minerals, or essential nutrients. Norman Jolliffe, MD, director of the Bureau of Nutrition at the New York Department of Health, now referred to sugar, fats, and oils in this manner. Jolliffe, as mentioned, founded a famous Manhattan weight-loss clinic and was author of the best-selling *Reduce and Stay Reduced*. He said that 35 percent of the calories Americans purchased were "empty." And, he added, deplorable.

In particular, Jolliffe despised highly caloric soft drinks. He was a great proponent of water as a beverage, but realistic enough to also support the new low-calorie sodas, as well as artificially sweetened iced tea and coffee. Other experts, including Fredrick J. Stare, director of nutrition for Harvard University's School of Public Health, seemingly disagreed with the position that sugar should be eliminated from the diet. In 1951, speaking to food writers at a luncheon paid for by the Sugar Research Foundation, Stare stressed that although the "core" of a good diet centered on milk products, meat, fish, eggs, fruits, vegetables, and whole grain or enriched products, there were a lot of options. "For example, one can drink one's milk as milk, in ice cream, or in the yogurt that is so much discussed," he said. Although he also stated that "obesity and dental caries are the most serious nutritional diseases afflicting adult Americans," he neglected to mention that consuming less sugar might be a preventive measure. The scientific director of the Sugar Research Foundation also spoke at the luncheon, explaining that food was more than just nutrients and fuel. What people ate was wrapped up in emotion, social activities, and religion. It was complicated, he said, suggesting that reducing sugar intake could be psychologically harmful. After all, who would even *think* about taking candy from a baby?

SWEETENING THE POT FOR ACADEMIA

Stare, who surely didn't believe this, did nothing to turn the argument around then or in the future, which is perhaps not surprising since he was best known for his incredible fund-raising abilities. In a few years, General Foods would give Harvard $1 million, at the time the largest gift ever made by a corporation, for the university to study obesity and heart disease. It is extremely possible that this was his motivation for lending his impressive title to the Sugar Research Foundation, whose primary goal was to promote the illusion that sugar was part of a healthy life.

In 1975 Stare coauthored a book with conservative medical writer Elizabeth Whelan, PhD. *Panic in the Pantry* is a political food manifesto that might have been cowritten by the CEOs of Domino, Dow, and Monsanto in response to slowly but steadily increasing suspicions about the

101

food supply in America. Rachel Carson's *Silent Spring*, published more than a decade earlier, was still widely read. Nutritionist Adelle Davis's series of books advocating unprocessed, natural foods free of hormones, antibiotics, and chemical additives (*Let's Eat Right to Keep Fit, Let's Get Well, Let's Cook It Right,* and *Let's Have Healthy Children*) had sold 7 million copies by the end of 1972. *Time* magazine called Davis "the high priestess of a new nutrition religion." Stare and Whelan suggested that readers should stop worrying about destroying the planet and what they served for dinner, and, most of all, stop fearing artificially sweetened foods as well as "good old natural sugar." Eating is supposed to be *fun,* the two experts in nutrition agreed, but "who could relax with a chilled Manhattan cocktail—or a bubbling diet soft drink—while glaring into the glass wondering if the maraschino cherry or the artificial sweetener was going to make him a cancer victim?" Stare and Whelan took the position that it was "unclear" whether artificial sweeteners were carcinogenic, and they were probably correct. But they also refuted any link between natural sweeteners and diabetes, tooth decay, coronary heart disease, obesity, or hypoglycemia, contrary to what "food faddists" or the tobacco industry (which was at that time busy blaming heart disease on anything but cigarettes) might want people to believe. "Sugar is an important source of energy," they emphatically stated, and "a most efficient product in terms of land use." Furthermore, they said, "Sugar is *not* a cause of diabetes, although high levels of sugar consumption may exacerbate the disease. . . . As to any relationship between sugar and coronary heart disease, there is really no basis for concern." Food is fun, so eat, drink, and be merry, said the chairman of Harvard's Department of Public Health and his protégée. Well, not exactly. As they put it: "Eat, drink and be *wary* of those who raise questions about the safety of your food."

DOES SUGAR CONTRIBUTE TO HEART DISEASE?

Many leading nutritionists, including the chairman of the home economics department at the University of California at Berkeley, agreed that excessive sugar in the diet was a leading factor in tooth decay, as well as a possible contributing factor in other diseases. John Yudkin, MD, who founded the department of nutrition at Queen Elizabeth College in London, argued in the British medical journal *The Lancet* that sugar was as likely to be responsible for obesity and heart disease as fat was. After completing a comparative study of 41 nations, he concluded that it was impossible to distinguish the negative impact of fat from that of sugar—wealthy populations consumed too much of both—and many highly caloric foods were a combination of the two. He felt it was therefore illogical to ignore the role sugar might play in diabetes, heart disease, and, of course, obesity.

Ancel Keys, PhD, of the University of Minnesota, convinced that saturated fat, not sugar, was the cause of coronary heart disease, argued that Yudkin had selected only countries that supported his thesis and "conveniently omitted" Venezuela and Cuba, where diets were high in sugar but the incidence of heart attacks was nevertheless "notably low." Keys believed there was no conclusive evidence that a diet low in sugar would reduce the frequency of heart attacks.

Many scientists, however, were questioning the health effects of sugar consumption. Even Keys said he deplored the fact that people were consuming so much of it (Americans at that time took in more than 20 percent of their calories as sugar), and there was no mistaking its role in obesity. Yudkin continued to publish research results throughout the 1960s that connected sugar to heart disease. Most of this was animal research, but in one study college students fed a high-sugar diet developed raised blood levels of cholesterol, triglycerides, and insulin, along with stickier blood cells that Yudkin thought might explain the clots that often were precursors of heart attacks. In 1972 he published *Pure, White and Deadly*, but the public and the scientific community had stopped listening.

It was difficult to convince people not to eat pure, white sugar, especially since the sugar industry's massive advertising budget made certain that controversy surrounded the issue of sucrose and health. The sugar lobby also had tremendous power on both sides of the aisle on Capitol Hill, and reputable men like Fredrick Stare continued to defend it as part of a healthy diet. Fat, on the other hand, was about to be irrevocably vilified as the main and only cause of coronary disease. *Maybe* sugar would result in a cavity. *Maybe* you would put on a few pounds. *Maybe* it could combine with fat and cause a little harm. But fat, on the other hand, could cost you your life. "Fat"—even its name implies bad things. Roses are red, violets are blue, sugar is sweet, and fat is a lumpy, unappealing serial killer.

FEAR OF FAT

In the early 1950s, evidence that too much fat was bad for your heart (along with your waistline) was accumulating, especially after a 1953 Harvard study linked cholesterol to arteriosclerosis. In 1954, specialists from the United States, Italy, northern Europe, Japan, South Africa, and Iraq concurred that a high-fat diet was linked to hardening of the arteries, and that the United States had the highest death rate in the world from cardiovascular disease. It was mentioned that in this one way, if in little else, underprivileged countries had the advantage over wealthier nations because there was so little fat in their diets. At a week-long meeting of the American Chemical Society, Keys argued that calories didn't cause heart disease: Dietary fat—specifically cholesterol—was the culprit.*

Heart health became headline news in 1955, when Lyndon Johnson, then the 46-year-old, 6-foot-3-inch, 200-pound Senate majority leader from Texas, had a heart attack. Zephyr Wright, his cook for more than 20 years, told the press that the senator loved his chocolate soufflé, ice cream, spoon bread, popovers, and tapioca pudding, which, sadly, she wasn't allowed to serve him anymore. In September, columnist Ida Jean Kain interviewed Johnson, who claimed that he was demanding a daily memo from his cook listing the number of fat grams in absolutely everything he ate. He had lost almost 20 pounds, he said, on his new, low-cholesterol diet. No butter or egg yolks for him.

Johnson had barely been discharged from the hospital when President Dwight D. Eisenhower suffered a heart attack right after eating a

---

* For further discussion about Keys's establishing cholesterol as solitary villain, see: Susan Allport, *The Queen of Fats* (Berkeley, CA: University of California Press, 2006).

hamburger. Television made information about his illness and recovery widely available, and he wisely made the decision to be open about his situation, successfully calming a fearful nation. Boston heart specialist Paul Dudley White, friend of both Vilhjalmur Stefansson and Keys and Eisenhower's head physician, was frequently interviewed about the president's condition and his new "low-fat" meal plan.

The country was getting an education in heart disease and nutrition. Prior to the attack, White said, Eisenhower followed a "typical" American diet, which in the 1950s meant that 40 percent of his daily calories were from fat, while the optimal amount was 30 percent, which had been "typical" in the 1930s. A connection between dietary fat and heart disease was more than just implied; White said it was "strongly suspected."

Cigarettes were also beginning to be "strongly suspected" of contributing to a high risk of coronary death. In September 1955, a medical study conclusively established a connection between the two, but fat still managed to play a part in that report, which stated that high levels of body fat correlated to high mortality and that male smokers had larger fat particles in their blood than nonsmokers. What this meant was unclear, but who wanted big fat particles coursing through their veins?

Jolliffe presented a paper stating that increased consumption of *both* fat and sugar were of significance in the frequency of degenerative heart disease, and that the important thing was for weight to be in the normal range. However, he said it would be better for a man to stay on a low-fat diet and remain overweight than to lose weight, regain it, and lose it again. Implicit in this statement is that remaining overweight on a low-fat diet could be accomplished only by eating a tremendous amount of carbohydrates, and in the following year, even Jolliffe changed course and made fat his solitary macronutrient villain. "No prudent person who has had, or wishes to avoid, coronary heart disease should eat a high-fat diet consumed by most Americans. This applies to all races and occupations, to the physically active and the sedentary, from the chain-smoking, tense, ambitious executive to the satisfied, relaxed barkeeper." Jolliffe, like Keys, became fat specific (saturated was bad, unsaturated was good), but not carbohydrate specific like Yudkin (sugar is bad, all other carbohydrates are good), and his conclusion was startling. "Stress and strain, physical indolence, obesity, luxury living or tobacco play but a minor role in producing a high coronary heart disease rate under 65 years of age, unless a high intake of saturated fat is added to these factors."

Without question, scientists like Jolliffe, White, and Keys were making huge contributions to health by focusing the public's attention on the correlation between diet and disease. However, the disagreement over what caused heart disease and obesity continued. Some experts, like Howard Burchell, MD, professor of medicine at the Mayo Foundation Graduate School of the University of Minnesota in Rochester, warned that making a revolutionary change in eating habits based on the available evidence was not justified. He believed that not enough was yet understood and that the research methods used might have been flawed. Keys, also at the University of Minnesota, remained adamant that low blood cholesterol levels were linked to a low frequency of coronary heart disease and that the meat and dairy fats in the American diet raised cholesterol while unsaturated fats like those in vegetable oils lowered it. Yudkin continued to argue that sugar should not be exonerated, for it too could be implicated in heart disease and was perhaps even the real and only culprit. Because Jolliffe had reversed his position, it seemed that no one thought *both* sugar and saturated fat might be a problem.

If the most highly respected experts in the world disagreed, it is understandable that nonexperts would remain, once again, confused. Obesity was unattractive, but was it dangerous? If certain fats help your heart but hurt your waistline, what are you supposed to eat?

If only someone could explain exactly what to eat and separate fact from fad. Actually, what to eat had been revealed and was widely available since *Diet and Health, with Key to the Calories* had become a bestseller. Norman Jolliffe's *Reduce and Stay Reduced* was also filled with good advice. It was just so damn boring.

10

DIETING BY THE BOOK

IN THE EARLY 1950S, WEIGHT-LOSS COOKBOOKS OFFERED STERN, CALORIE-RESTRICTIVE plans and had unexciting titles like *Reducer's Cook Book, Reducing Cookbook and Diet Guide,* and *The Low-Calory Cookbook.*

The Low-Calory Cookbook lives up to its title. The introduction by Donald Armstrong (of none other than the Metropolitan Life Insurance Company) gets right to the point: 25 million people in the United States are overweight, and the time to reduce is now. The cookbook's author, Bernard Koten, describes himself as "just a guy interested in good eating," who, after reaching 250 pounds, found an effective way to reduce at Norman Jolliffe's weight-loss clinic. (This was 9 years before Jean Nidetch went there and devised a way to make the information interesting.)

Koten says he is a great admirer of Jolliffe and dedicates the book to him, but he also says that Jolliffe's plan is "rigid and unappetizing." Ironically, what follows is a group of rigid and unappetizing recipes. No sugar, starch, or fat is allowed; his diet is actually far more stringent than Jolliffe's. A recipe for Creamed Chicken calls for toasting a cup of powdered skimmed milk with salt over low heat until it turns brown, adding a cup of liquid skim milk, stirring them together until smooth, then adding a cup of cooked, skinless chicken, along with some parsley, pimento, and paprika—a concoction that surely wouldn't go into a beloved family recipes file. To complete the meal, Fruit Bavarian is a mere 50 calories' worth of chilled powdered gelatin mixed with skimmed milk, water-packed canned fruit, salt, lemon juice, and 40 (you had to count them) tiny grains of saccharin crystals. This could be topped with Whipped Cream, the ingredients for which were skim milk, gelatin, water, vanilla, and 15 grains of saccharin crystals.

Jolliffe's *Reduce and Stay Reduced* had fewer recipes (his version of Whipped Topping, by the way, is a combination of water, lemon juice, vanilla, fat-free milk powder, and granulated sugar) and is essentially a volume of charts, meal plans, and instructions on how to eat well while doing what the title promises, along with extensive lists of "calorie counts" for common foods. For example, there are lists of all-you-can-eat foods that have zero calories (black coffee, tea, seltzer, spices, vinegar, dill pickles, clear soups, lemon juice); vegetables that are *almost* all-you-can-eat because they have only $12\frac{1}{2}$ calories per $\frac{1}{2}$ cup, which are referred to as "$12\frac{1}{2}$-Calorie-Count" vegetables (mushrooms, broccoli, and lettuce); vegetables that are "25-Calorie-Count" (carrots, eggplant); "50-Calorie-Count" (parsnips, squash); etc. The same types of lists are provided for various calorie counts of fruits. Meat, fish, poultry, breads and crackers, dairy foods, cereals, desserts, and beverages—including alcohol—are all assigned numbers. This is a terrific plan for motivated people—learn the caloric and nutritive values of various foods, establish a daily calorie budget, and stay well within its parameters. It's an approach that's similar to the one taken by several popular weight-loss plans today—including Nidetch's Weight Watchers. She simplified the charts, but other than that, her original Weight Watchers diet differs very little from Jolliffe's plan. She just made it more fun.

SLOW FOOD NATION OF TWO

On January 13, 1961, 57-year-old anticholesterol advocate Ancel Keys was the man on the cover of *Time* magazine. Most people probably wouldn't recognize his name today, which is not surprising; scientists rarely achieve lasting fame unless their names are attached to products or inventions. If the Mediterranean Diet were called the Keys Diet, we would remember him for introducing that delightfully healthful way of eating to America. If the lightweight, easy-to-carry, nutritious meals he developed for paratroopers and field soldiers during World War II were known as Keys rations instead of just K rations, that might also have resulted in name recognition. Luckily, Keys didn't seem to care much whether or not people knew his name. His daughter Carrie once described him as a humble man who wanted people to look at his research, but not at him.

Born in Colorado Springs in 1904, Keys's life was peripatetic from the start. When he was a baby, his teenaged parents moved to Berkeley, California, to look for work, then on to Los Angeles as refugees after the 1906 San Francisco earthquake, then back to Berkeley once more. When Ancel was 15, he left home for a job shoveling bat manure from a cave in Oatman, Arizona, and then went on to work in a Colorado gold mine. When he returned, he finished high school and enrolled at the University of California, Berkeley, as a chemistry major. But before completing his undergraduate degree, he signed up to work on an oil freighter headed for China. The sailors' diet, he later said, was composed mostly of alcohol.

When he returned to Berkeley, he made a surprising switch in his field of study from chemistry to economics, and after he graduated, he went to work for F. W. Woolworth and Company. His career with the discount retailer was brief; after 8 months, intolerably bored, Keys returned to Berkeley, where he would complete a doctoral degree in biology in 3 years. For the rest of his life, he followed this odd but predictable pattern of engaging in intense intellectual activity followed by periods of exotic travel and adventure. And sometimes, both of these worlds would combine.

In the years that followed his doctoral work, Keys studied under 1920 Nobel laureate biochemist August Krogh in Copenhagen; acquired an additional PhD in physiology at Cambridge; spent time on an 18,000-foot mountain peak in the Chilean Andes while studying the effects of high altitude on miners (as part of a Harvard study); and went to work for the Mayo Clinic at the University of Minnesota, where he found a more or less permanent home and a woman with whom to have an enduring marriage.

In 1939, at the age of 35, he founded the Laboratory of Physiological Hygiene at the University of Minnesota's School of Public Health and remained its director for 33 years. His landmark Minnesota Experiment, which analyzed the psychological as well as the physiological effects of human starvation, was completed there. This is where his classic textbook *The Biology of Human Starvation* was written, and where he developed his groundbreaking predictive equations that were intended to discern, as he would phrase it, why people got sick *before* they got sick. This is where the numbers were crunched on thousands of blood serum cholesterol samples he and his team had gathered from all over the world. He was the director of an interdisciplinary, egalitarian environment where biologists, anthropologists, physiologists, psychologists, and biochemists shared ideas. Tea was served at 3:30 p.m. every afternoon and all were invited, including clerical and custodial staff.

Keys's curriculum vitae was so impressive that items of great distinction—he was, for example, a senior Fulbright fellow at Oxford—might be omitted for lack of space. However, it was during this sabbatical at Oxford in 1950 that he and his wife Margaret, a biochemist and one of his primary researchers, were informed by a colleague that there was very little heart disease among the population of southern Italy. Intrigued, he and Margaret traveled to Naples, where they discovered that the serum cholesterol levels in the blood of the Italian firefighters and city employees they tested were very low, in contrast to that of a comparable socioeconomic group in Minnesota: 165 milligrams per deciliter versus 230. Neapolitan coronary heart disease patients were rare. When they tested cholesterol levels of wealthier Italians who consumed richer diets, the results were more similar to, but still better than, those of the Americans. They write about this "common folks diet" in the 1975 book *How to Eat Well and Stay Well the Mediterranean Way,* in which they detail a diet that includes homemade minestrone; pasta with sauce, grated cheese, and perhaps a bit of meat; pasta fagioli; bread warm from the oven; lots of fresh, seasonal vegetables; small portions of meat or fish once or twice a week; fruit for dessert; and red wine. With recipe variations for cuisines from other countries, such as Spanish paella and Greek moussaka, this philosophy of eating lots of fruits and vegetables in season, along with whole grains, breads, cheeses, and small amounts of meat and fish, became the Keyses' Mediterranean diet. It was essentially an international version of their popular 1959 cookbook, *Eat Well and Stay Well*, which presented seasonal recipes and menus low in saturated fats ("Remember that rich foods are essential only to bad cooks," Margaret admonishes) and recommended fresh foods (local if possible) consumed respectfully and slowly. In 1966, Roy de Groot would write *Feasts for All Seasons*, which had a similar message and excellent recipes. All three cookbooks stressed taking a healthier approach to mealtime along with moderation and enjoyment of a variety of fresh foods, and all are quite similar to de Groot's original Rockefeller Diet.

The Keyses' research in Naples led to the monumental Seven Countries Study of 12,000 healthy, middle-aged men from rural areas in Italy, Greece, Yugoslavia, Holland, Finland, Japan, and the United States. The results strongly supported the link between coronary heart disease and a diet high in saturated fat. The diets of the participants in Finland and the United States were highest in saturated fat ("They put butter on slabs of cheese in Finland," Keys said), and those of the Japanese were lowest. Ironically, the Seven Countries Study also measured sugar consumption, and it too appeared to be a predictor of heart disease. But Keys chose to focus only on fat. Heart disease correlated with high cholesterol, and that's what became headline news. This is why most Americans today, even if they know little else about their health statistics, know their cholesterol levels. And it's also why Keys appeared on the cover of *Time* magazine.

Keys wrote hundreds of academic articles and books throughout his career. With his wife, Margaret, he wrote two best-selling Mediterranean-diet cookbooks, as well as a third called *The Benevolent Bean*. The royalties from their book sales enabled the couple to build a home in a little seaside village south of Naples, with a garden and a small grove of fruit trees also on the property. It was where they spent most of their time after they left academia in 1972.

Keys, who weighed 155 pounds and was 5 feet 7½ inches tall, said his daily breakfast consisted of half a grapefruit, dry cereal with skim milk, unbuttered toast, jam, and coffee. He brown-bagged his lunch, usually a sardine sandwich, olives, a cookie, and a glass of skim milk. Meals should be eaten with "deliberate slowness," he said, because "I don't like to insult food." Dinner was a romantic and relaxing ritual with Margaret, who concocted and tested all of the recipes in their cookbooks. She rarely served the same dish within a 3-week period. Their dinners lasted for up to 2 hours and included classical music, candlelight, multiple courses, and a predinner cocktail (a martini or negroni). The 1,000-calorie meal that followed consisted of no more than 20 percent fats of any kind. A sample menu includes: pasta al brodo (turkey broth with noodles), veal scallopini à la Marsala, fresh green beans, a tossed salad with vinaigrette dressing, homemade bread, cookies, espresso, and fruit. A "carving meat," like a roast, might be served as often as three times a week.

The Keyses' respect for and enjoyment of food is evident. They were not trying to be the food police, nor were they gluttons. Margaret, who was often said to have a calming effect on her cyclone of a husband, was a scientist, writer, researcher, and mother. And still, she baked her own bread, tested new recipes, and prepared multicourse meals nightly.

They continued to enjoy this productive and civilized life until 2004, when Ancel died at the age of 100. He was still publishing until 2001. Margaret died in 2006, at the age of 97.

11

EAT FAT, GET THIN

IN THE SAME YEAR THAT ANCEL KEYS APPEARED ON THE COVER OF *TIME* AND ALMOST 100 years after William Banting printed his *Letter on Corpulence, Addressed to the Public,* Romanian-born gynecologist Herman Taller, MD, presented a weight-loss theory in his book, *Calories Don't Count,* that he claimed was "revolutionary." The book was not quite that innovative, but it certainly was unusual. Taller's low-carbohydrate, very-high-fat diet was based on his bizarre theory that you could eat 5,000 calories a day as long as you included 3 ounces of safflower oil with every meal, even if you drank it by the glass. (Keys wrote that some farmers on Crete begin each day by drinking a wine glass full of olive oil, although that's where any similarity between the Mediterranean diet and Taller's plan ended. Vilhjalmur Stefansson also noted the wonders of oil, describing Scandinavian fishermen who regarded cod or halibut liver oil as "nearly magical," often drinking a glassful of it in the morning.)

Taller's book was a haphazard collection of bits of information that acknowledged as antecedents no one except Alfred Pennington, who had become so well known because of the Holiday Diet that it was impossible for Taller to ignore him. The absurd recommendation of a 5,000-calorie-a-day diet was likely lifted from Stefansson, who had written that an all-meat diet should be 80 percent fat and 20 percent lean and that if one bought 1,000 calories' worth of lean meat, the butcher would gladly give 4,000 calories' worth of fat along with it for free. Stefansson had never suggested that the entire purchase should be consumed in 1 day. The safflower oil idea probably came from an experiment financed by the food conglomerate Unilever in the

113

mid-1950s that tested the benefits of a vitamin A–fortified safflower margarine. Subjects at Texas State College for Women who were put on moderately high-fat (30 to 35 percent) diets lost weight *and* gained clearer complexions when they ate the vitamin-enriched spread.

None of this had anything to do with safflower oil, but that's what Taller was selling. If you found the stuff unpalatable, he said, simply order easy-to-swallow pills from Cove Vitamin and Pharmaceutical of Glen Cove, Long Island. Take two before every meal.

Taller claimed that his "entirely safe and entirely effective" diet was tested successfully not only on himself, but on large numbers of patients in medical laboratories and, amazingly, there were no failures. He stated that the scientific research backing his breakthrough had been published in numerous journals, although he cited none of them. "I would no more offer an untested program to the public than I would offer an untested program to a patient who walked into my office filled with faith that I would do the right thing to the best of my ability and knowledge," he wrote in his introduction.

Taller said that the reason his diet worked was that the body can burn unlimited fat, but only a finite amount of carbohydrates, and he reminded his readers that salads and fruits are carbohydrates, too, and thus should be avoided. He also suggested that for a woman, losing weight could lead to an all-around better life, resulting in more energy for housework and other, more romantic benefits. "An obese woman in a messy house is not the average man's ideal of marriage," he said, absurdly defining obese as even 1 or 2 pounds more than the Metropolitan Life Insurance Company's new ideal-weight charts and neglecting to mention that a fat man in a messy house might not be a woman's fantasy either. Ironically, Taller denounced fads. He despised pills, powders, and exercising machines. "Mankind seems to have a natural weakness for food fads," he concluded.

Calories Don't Count became a bestseller, remaining near the top of the list even after the New York office of the FDA seized 1,600 copies of it along with 58,000 safflower seed oil capsules the following January. One capsule supplied 5½ grams, or about 50 calories, of safflower oil daily, which the FDA described as "insignificant for any purpose." In other words, those six pills a day would not result in lower cholesterol, increased sexual desire, a better complexion, and a stronger heart or spell the end of heartburn and the common cold as it also helped you lose weight fast. The FDA ruled that all of Taller's claims were "false and misleading." Undaunted, publisher Simon and Schuster continued to run full-page advertisements promoting the bestseller.

In July, George P. Larrick, commissioner of the FDA, charged that *Calories Don't Count* was "deliberately created and used to promote sales of 'worthless safflower oil capsules.'" In a front-page story, the *New York Times* reported that Simon and Schuster denounced the charge as "vicious and irresponsible." Commissioner Larrick argued that although freedom to publish a "health book" was a constitutional right, if that book used false statements and claims to promote a pharmaceutical product, it fell under the jurisdiction of the FDA. This was Taller's critical mistake. If his book had simply made wildly inaccurate statements about health and weight loss, it would have been just another entry on a long list of bestsellers full of dubious weight-loss advice. He would have been rich, and not under indictment.

According to Larrick, Simon and Schuster admitted that the first draft of Taller's manuscript had been "too scientific." Roger Kahn, a freelance writer, had been hired to revise it "in a more mail-order inspirational technique." Kahn, who would later be lauded as one of the great sportswriters of all time, had come up with the brilliant title. The manuscript then went to the office of the General Development Corporation, a Florida land development firm, for the "purpose of inserting references" to safflower oil pills. The CDC (for Calories Don't Count) Corporation was established as a division of Cove Vitamin and Pharmaceutical to manufacture and distribute the pills. The financial interests of CDC were acquired by Taller, two executives at Simon and Schuster, officials of the General Development Corporation, and Cove Vitamin and Pharmaceutical. "The plain fact is weight reduction requires the reduction of caloric intake," Larrick concluded, not 5,000 calories a day and oil pills.

Cove sued Simon and Schuster for $6.5 million on grounds that an agreement between the two to market the capsules along with the book had been broken. Simon and Schuster countersued Cove for $7.5 million for copyright infringement, stating that *Calories Don't Count* had been used to promote the sale of the capsules, a relationship that the publisher had never sanctioned. By the end of the month, Taller's book was still number three on the *New York Times* nonfiction bestseller list. More than 1 million copies had been sold.

In March 1964, a federal grand jury in Brooklyn indicted Herman Taller. "If convicted, pudgy Taller faces a maximum of 239 years of good, starchy prison fare," *Time* magazine inaccurately gloated. In 1967, the 56-year-old doctor, depicted by the *New York Times* as an "urbane native of Rumania" who "took the verdict calmly," was found guilty of 12 counts of mail fraud, conspiracy, and violating federal drug regulations, but innocent of 37 other charges. In actuality, he faced a maximum of 50 years in prison and $71,000 in fines, but his sentence was lenient, a fine of $7,000 and 2 years' probation. He served no jail time; all of the other counts were suspended, and his medical license was revoked.

Many American dieters, in the meantime, had found something even better than eating all the steak and safflower oil they wanted: having a martini before the meal and a glass of wine with it.

BELLY UP TO THE BAR, BOYS

Robert Cameron was a cosmetics executive in New York City when he decided he had taken one commuter train ride too many and moved his family to San Francisco, which, he liked to say, was a much simpler move than the one his mother had made when she went from Cincinnati to Iowa in a Conestoga wagon. A charming man with far-left political leanings, Cameron loved socializing—especially with a cocktail in hand (preferably a martini or gimlet). San Francisco was just his sort of town, and he settled in, made friends, and was struck with a great idea: a weight-loss diet that included alcohol, something a bit more palatable to the "100 million people in the country who have a drink now and then."

If there were a prize for the most irresistible diet-book title of all time, Cameron might win. In 1964 he self-published *The Drinking Man's Diet*, selling his 60-page, 4- by 7-inch booklet for $1. There had been nothing quite like it since Banting's *Letter on Corpulence,* which itself had been self-published at a time when alcohol was believed to have no calories. (Sorry, it does.) Cameron suggested that alcohol had calories but no carbohydrates and therefore was an acceptable diet food. His eating plan—a variation on a popular diet created by the US Air Force —was predicated on the idea that calories *do* count, but are not created equal. Because fats have a high satiety value, they were "good" calories, while carbohydrates were just the opposite. Essentially, it was Herman Taller's plan without oil by the glassful. Or, for that matter, a variation of many other popular diets that had preceded Cameron's, except that you could drink a lot. He sold 2.4 million books within about a year.

Cameron realistically stated: "If you gorge yourself with food, even if it is low in carbohydrates, you will get fat. If you drink too much you will get drunk." Nevertheless, this diet is high in animal fat and very low in carbohydrates, and *not* drinking too much can mean a martini or highball before lunch and/or dinner, as well as two glasses of wine with each meal "if desired," although he reminds followers that they don't *have* to drink to lose weight. Nutritionists were outraged, perhaps even more so than usual, because of the cavalier approach to alcohol consumption in a generation only once removed from Prohibition. Fredrick Stare, who had stated in his introductory comments to his friend Stefansson's *Fat of the Land,* "One of the most interesting developments of modern nutrition has been the emergence of a number of studies emphasizing the great ability of experimental animals, including man, to adapt to wide variations in diet," predicted that this fad would soon be over. Theodore B. VanItallie, MD, of New York's St. Luke's Hospital called it "a passing fad like the yo-yo or hula hoop, and about as worthwhile," and Jean Mayer, PhD, of Harvard ominously said it was "in a sense equivalent to mass murder." It was the latter comment that caused sales of the book to plummet, but Cameron had already made a small fortune, which allowed him to follow his passion. Strapped into a helicopter with the door removed, his first aerial photo-essay, *Above San Francisco,* accompanied by text from well-known San Francisco columnist Herb Caen, was a success. Cameron went on to publish many other books in a series, including *Above Paris* with Pierre Salinger and *Above London* with

Alistair Cooke. In 2004, at the age of 93, he released *Above Mexico City* and rereleased *The Drinking Man's Diet*, and 2 years later he invited 150 of his closest friends to celebrate his 95th birthday and have a drink. Cameron died in 2009 at the age of 98. Three months earlier he had photographed his beloved San Francisco from a helicopter for the last time.

DO YOU BELIEVE IN MIRACLES?

Irwin Maxwell Stillman, MD, was a family doctor in Brooklyn for 45 years before retiring to Florida in 1967 and writing *The Doctor's Quick Weight Loss Diet* with Samm Sinclair Baker, a prolific copywriter and advertising executive turned author. The diet was said to be "medically proven" based on Stillman's personal experience as a physician and Baker's personal experience as a dieter, and it did, in fact, work. How could it not? It was, after all, a high-protein, no-fat, no-carbohydrate diet.

Stillman claimed a bonus 275 calories would be burned daily as long as you ate only from his "extensive" list of high-protein foods and *nothing else*. He warned that even a piece of chewing gum or a piece of hard candy might result in failure. The list was short and to the point:

- Lean meat, trimmed of all fat, broiled or boiled
- Chicken or turkey, no skin, broiled
- Lean fish, such as flounder or cod, broiled
- Seafood, such as shrimp or scallops, broiled
- Eggs, hard-boiled or fried in a nonstick pan without oil
- Fat-free milk
- Cottage cheese
- Black coffee, tea, club soda, and diet soda
- Salt, pepper, garlic, and ketchup
- Eight glasses of water a day (mandatory)

No other foods were permissible, including fruits, vegetables, pasta, bread, rice, or fats. It was suggested that you test yourself daily for ketones (via a urine sample) to establish that you weren't cheating and that the diet was working correctly. This is why 8 glasses of water a day were mandatory; otherwise the strain on the kidneys might be devastating if you were in a state of ketosis. It is also the reason why people on any type of very-low-carbohydrate diet are initially so happy with the results—weight loss occurs quickly as a result of eating fewer calories combined with water loss. (The elevated ketones are also responsible for the noticeable breath odor, akin to nail polish remover, of many low-carb dieters.)

Stillman recommended that a 5-foot-4-inch female, dressed but without jacket or shoes, should "ideally" weigh a diminutive 108 pounds. According to the Metropolitan Life weight charts of the time, the "ideal" weight for a female of that height with a small frame was 108 to 116 pounds, which went up to 138 pounds for a woman with a large frame (with her shoes on). Stillman had even more stringent standards for women who were models, actresses, dancers, or athletes, recommending they lose an *additional* 5 pounds, which sounds suspiciously like the making of an anorexic at a time when the paper-thin British model Twiggy had became popular in America. His "desirable" weights were the lowest ever published, paradoxically at a time when an actual rather than perceived obesity epidemic was about to begin.

It was necessary to follow Stillman's all-protein starvation plan until you lost 30 pounds, at which time you were able to add yogurt, artificially sweetened gelatin, vegetables, fruits, bread, honey, and jam back into your diet. But you still had to be vigilant—if you gained back more than 3 pounds, you had to go back to the beginning.

If you didn't want to count calories or return to the all-protein plan, Stillman offered other methods, including fasting for 1 to 2 days a week *for the rest of your life*, a "semi-starvation" diet consisting of one hard-boiled egg, 8 ounces of skim milk, 3½ ounces of salad without dressing, and 8 glasses of water for as long as you could take it, or a 40-calorie-a-day diet of lettuce leaves and tomato slices with black coffee and 8 glasses of water. There was a buttermilk diet—6 glasses a day and nothing else—or the all-meat option of ½ pound of meat three times a day, which was what Stefansson and Anderson ate during their yearlong experiment. It was as if Stillman and Baker had cataloged every insane weight-loss fad of the past 50 years; they even brought back the bananas and skim milk fad of the 1930s.

Stillman's book sold millions of copies. It was followed by a cookbook and three other weight-loss titles, and his program became one of America's first diet-book franchises. It might even have rivaled *Dr. Atkins' Diet Revolution*, first published in 1972, except that Irwin Maxwell Stillman died of a heart attack in 1975, leaving Baker to search for another doctor with a scheme.

THE SINGLE MAN'S DIET

Wealthy and sophisticated bachelor Herman Tarnower, MD, was a perfect match for Baker—and a perfect catch for women. He was a Scarsdale, New York, cardiologist, a popular member of Westchester County society, and very different from Irwin Stillman, the quiet family man and general practitioner from Brooklyn. Tarnower lived on an estate in Westchester County, New York, where he gave frequent and elegant dinner parties catered by a Frenchwoman whose landscape-gardener husband grew the fresh herbs and luscious vegetables she prepared. *New York Times* food writer Craig Claiborne was a guest in 1979 and gave excellent reviews to the "impressive" wines, "insidiously tempting" fried cheese and anchovy toast, salmon mousse made with fish netted by the host himself on a recent fly-fishing expedition, boneless chicken breasts in a Madeira and raisin sauce, zucchini from the garden in a light cream sauce, and, for dessert, a concoction of apples, whipped cream, and macadamia nuts. "The important thing in dieting," Tarnower tells Claiborne, "is to eat in moderation." Eating good food but not too much of it was not advice that could be stretched into a best-selling book even by an expert like Baker, however. For that, it was necessary to develop yet one more variation of "eat less" masquerading as something revolutionary. Tarnower had been handing out mimeographed copies of a semi-low-carbohydrate plan for years, he said in the introduction to *The Complete Scarsdale Medical Diet Plus Dr. Tarnower's Lifetime Keep-Slim Program.* This is a sample of the original meal plan for Thursday:

> Breakfast: (the same each day) ½ grapefruit, 1 slice protein bread without spread, coffee or tea with no milk

Lunch: cold chicken, raw or cooked spinach, coffee or tea

Dinner: 2 eggs any style but prepared without any fat, cottage cheese, cooked cabbage, 1 slice protein toast without spread, coffee or tea

Herman Tarnower wrote that he'd never intended to distribute his diet to anyone but patients and friends, but a surprising surge in publicity resulted in letters and phone calls from thousands of people requesting more information. And so, he made his wisdom available to all.

All of this "surprising" publicity was actually the result of a $25,000 advertising campaign funded by Kennett Rawson of Rawson, Wade Publishing, who published the book, as well as *Dr. Atkins' Diet Revolution* in 1972. Rawson knew the potential of this type of fad diet, especially if it had a cardiologist behind it. Samm Sinclair Baker, the one-man bestseller factory, had been searching for Stillman's replacement for years and approached Tarnower, who readily agreed to a partnership. In 3 months they extended the original mimeographed pages into a 212-page book that was released in 1978. *The Complete Scarsdale Medical Diet*, which was in actuality just another low-calorie diet named after a fancy location, aimed high—it promised the loss of at least 14 pounds in 2 weeks. "We are geared to a fast-moving world, and programmed to need and expect fast results," Tarnower said in the introduction, explaining that the first 14 days were followed by a 14-day "keep-trim" program, during which you could enjoy a cocktail before dinner or a glass of wine with your meal. Then, after quickly attaining your goal, you simply needed to eat right forever and "keep trim." The worst-case scenario meant uncomfortably depriving yourself only half of the time, as your weight became an unhealthy series of valleys and peaks.

The method was simple: You followed a low-calorie meal plan exactly as written, choosing from the equally depressing and extremely similar Basic, Gourmet, Vegetarian, Money-Saver, and International diets. To be a "Scarsdale Loser and a Lifetime Winner" you also had to avoid second helpings, desserts, fried foods, and all between-meal snacks except carrots. And, reminiscent of Horace Fletcher's masticating advice, you had to chew your food thoroughly.

The bestseller would likely have been quickly replaced and forgotten if Herman Tarnower hadn't been shot dead by his 56-year-old female companion on March 11, 1980, a few days before his 70th birthday.

The murder became the subject of numerous books and two films. Jean Harris, the divorced headmistress of an exclusive prep school for girls and 1945 summa cum laude graduate of Smith College, had been Tarnower's faithful companion for many years and was said to be aware that he often strayed. Although *The Complete Scarsdale Medical Diet* is not dedicated to her (or anyone else), she is the first person thanked in the acknowledgments section for her "splendid assistance in the researching and writing of this book." Lynne Tryforos, a 37-year-old nurse at Tarnower's medical facility and his lover, is thanked further down the list. Tryforos was at the house the night Harris shot him four times.

On February 25, 1981, after a trial that caused the kind of media frenzy that only the problems of the rich and famous can arouse, Jean Harris was found guilty of second-degree murder and sentenced to 15 years in prison. She wrote three books and taught English classes to inmates before her 1992 pardon, and she currently resides in an assisted-living facility in Connecticut. Samm Sinclair Baker died in 1997, having written or coauthored more than 30 books, as well as three mysteries. His last diet book, coauthored in 1987, was *The Dr. DeBetz Champagne Diet*. Its gimmick was self-hypnosis along with an optional daily 3-ounce glass of the bubbly as a little luxury in an otherwise austere 1,200-calorie-a-day life.

At the time of his death, Herman Tarnower had just begun outlining a new book about how to achieve and enjoy longevity.

12

DON'T START THE REVOLUTION WITHOUT ATKINS

IN 1968 THE AMERICAN PUBLIC RECEIVED A SHOCKING BIT OF NEWS: MORE THAN 10 million citizens living in the best-fed country on Earth were, in fact, undernourished. The CBS documentary *Hunger in America* won an Emmy Award for revealing this fact, and it directly resulted in the establishment of the Senate Select Committee on Nutrition and Human Needs in 1968, with Senator George McGovern, Democrat from the agricultural state of South Dakota, as chairman. The first 4 years were devoted to solving the problems of hunger, but in 1973 McGovern announced that attention also had to be paid to the estimated 30 percent of the population who were overweight, because, he said, "the overweight consumer is the most unprotected of them all."

The hearings focused on shielding the overweight and obese from fad diets and other harmful schemes, including one of the newest additions to the weight-loss canon: cardiologist Robert C. Atkins, MD, and his book, *Dr. Atkins' Diet Revolution: The High Calorie Way to Stay Thin Forever*. McGovern and the committee considered Atkins's book to be, perhaps, the worst of the "worthless, fraudulent" bunch—and that was quite a statement.

Diet Revolution, which had recently been published and was selling

123

like forbidden hot cakes, was singled out because it recommended the unlimited intake of fats of all kinds, including animal fats such as meat, egg yolks, and cheese, as well as the elimination of all carbohydrates, including fruits and vegetables. (By the way, lumping sugar, whole grains, processed white flour, rice, pasta, fruits, and vegetables together under the umbrella of "carbohydrates" without regard to the significant nutritional differences of these foods has probably caused more harm and confusion over the years than any other piece of dietary advice.)

Senator Charles Percy of Illinois read into the Senate record a statement by Fredrick Stare that condemned Atkins's book as "nonsense," "dangerous," and charged that "the author . . . is guilty of malpractice," which was, once again, odd since Stare had once written that his friend Vilhjalmur Stefansson's all-meat diet was a viable alternative for a physically active person. Three experts testified about the dangers of following Atkins's diet. Karlis Adamsons, an obstetrician at Mount Sinai Hospital in New York City, was astonished that Atkins recommended his plan for pregnant women. "If I were a fetus, I would forbid my mother to go on such a diet," he said, citing the research findings on why such a dietary plan would endanger an unborn child. Theodore B. VanItallie, vice chairman of the American Medical Association (AMA), warned that if followed for a lifetime, as suggested, the Atkins eating plan would greatly increase the risk of developing heart disease. And the AMA chairman, C. E. Butterworth, MD, said, "The full impact of such a diet may not become apparent until many years later."

Of course, Butterworth could not have fully appreciated how right he was. The cardiologist's diet that had captured the nation's heart would remain popular for decades, reappearing every few years under the guise of a "new" or "revised" plan. It would, eventually, evolve into a massive, international brand and lifestyle. Currently, the Atkins International Web site strings many of America's favorite buzzwords together and suggests that you relax and let "sweet sexy science" work for you. (If you are curious about how living "La Vida Low Carb," as they call it, can be sweet and sexy, it's by purchasing a line of highly processed, artificially sweetened, not-all-that-low-carb foods. The "science" part results from embracing studies that support Atkins while ignoring ones that don't.)

When Robert Atkins, accompanied by his lawyer, testified before Congress on April 12, 1973, he denied the charges that his book was unscientific and dangerous, claiming as his defense the "common sense observation of every dieter that sugars and starches are fattening." Atkins, of course, excluded the credible studies of high-protein diets conducted by Vilhjalmur Stefansson, Blake Donaldson, and Alfred Pennington, probably to protect the "revolutionary" claim he tied to his highly lucrative plan. He may have been the main witch hunted in the McGovern hearings, but he also had the potential for becoming the richest.

The appeal Atkins had for dieters was simple: A heart doctor says it's okay to eat a juicy, well-marbled steak, followed by an ice cream sundae topped off with nuts and whipped cream for dessert every night of the week—all while losing weight! It's easy to see how such a plan would dethrone the spartan, sour, unsexy Stillman—Atkins was a *high*-calorie plan. At the time of his first book's publication, Atkins was an attractive, 42-year-old physician on the Upper East Side of Manhattan ministering to the wealthy and occasionally boldfaced names that he dropped throughout his first book, like actress Leslie Uggams and film producer David Brown. Before attending medical school, he had worked, briefly, as an entertainer. Articles about his diet had run in numerous women's magazines, including *Vogue* and *Cosmopolitan* (whose editor-in-chief was Brown's wife, Helen Gurley Brown), and the cardiologist claimed that in the 7 years before publishing his book, he had helped 10,000 overweight people with his "revolutionary" methods, which would mean about 4 every day, without ever taking a day off, while maintaining a practice as a cardiologist. The book, which was written with Ruth West Herwood, is dedicated to the dedicated, his once and future patients: "all the diet revolutionaries who are not content merely to follow their own diet, but who are dedicated to carrying the message of the diet revolution to the world which needs it."

It sounds eerily similar to cult indoctrination, and in a sense it was. After a decade of trauma—beloved leaders assassinated and the violently contested Vietnam War still being fought—many were open to exploring the counterintuitive. Hundreds of thousands of people spent a lot of money to give up their weekends and attend existentialism seminars like Werner Erhard's Erhard Seminars Training (EST) in the hope of transforming their mental outlooks and their lives. Atkins wisely took advantage of the public's suspicion and mistrust of authority and marketed his diet to an audience of people willing to believe in a glamorous doctor quixotically fighting the establishment. He told his readers repeatedly not to let *anyone*, including nutritionists, physicians, and loved ones, talk them out of eating as much fat as they desired. His message was that if you are willing to dine only at the very top of the food chain forever, you will lose weight and permanently keep it off, your cholesterol and triglyceride levels will go down, your depression will miraculously go away, and your energy will soar to an all-time high.

Millions went on "Atkins." His primary message was, and remains, that overweight is not caused by overeating, but by a mysterious "metabolic imbalance" that physicians and dietitians are unfamiliar with. His diet is "deliberately unbalanced." His patients don't count calories, they count carbs, and they lose weight effectively, he says, on days that begin with bacon and eggs and coffee with heavy cream, include a 5-ounce cheeseburger and a cup of loosely packed salad greens with mayonnaise dressing for lunch, and finish up with six scampi with two big lamb chops and another cup of dressed green salad followed by a "special" dessert made from artificial sweetener, eggs, and cheese for dinner. (If you are wondering how salad is included on a no-carbohydrate-of-any-kind diet, an average salad is a large handful of greens, and greens are made up of water, fiber, vitamins, and minerals. That's why they are so low in calories; the more water there is in a food, the fewer calories. Measure for yourself—one loosely packed cup is almost no salad at all and therefore almost no carbohydrates. Indeed, any very-low-calorie food is also low in fat, carbohydrates, and protein. Two and one-half cups of greens a day, which is what the "induction phase allows," is extremely limited in both nutrients and fiber, but the color does perk up that plate of meat, and Atkins acknowledges this '70s style, saying that the greens prevent the diet from becoming "an uncivilized drag.")

Robert Atkins preached to the converted, suggesting that counting calories never works and that mainstream medicine's lack of success in

126

the weight-loss arena had become conspicuous in an "increasingly sedentary society." He asked: "Why hasn't medicine spoken?" And answered: "Because of vast endowments poured into various departments of nutritional education at major universities by manufacturers of refined carbohydrate food stuffs." We are all victims, he continued, of carbohydrate poisoning and sugar addiction, now consuming more sugar in 2 weeks than we did in a year a couple of centuries ago. From 4 pounds a year in 1750 to 110 pounds a year in 1972—11 generations is not enough time to produce the genetic change that is necessary to deal with so much sugar.

There is truth in Atkins's philosophy about processed foods and sugar—they make you fat and cause a wide variety of other health problems. The Senate Select Committee on Nutrition and Human Needs was critical of Atkins because he didn't *just* advocate eliminating nutritionally bankrupt, "empty" carbohydrates—"Coke, cake, catsup, cookies and candy bars," as he put it. After the initial period of carbohydrate abstinence, only about 5 grams are restored to the daily diet each week, a number that is steadily increased until the dieter is no longer in a state of ketosis, and then reduced once more until ketosis becomes permanent. Ketosis is tested daily in the same way that Stillman recommended—if an Acetest tablet turns purple when it comes in contact with your urine, you are still in the game. For most people, this means only about 20 to 40 grams of carbohydrates per day; a medium apple has 21 grams. (The current USDA dietary recommendation is that carbohydrates should make up about 50 percent of your daily calories. On a 2,000-calorie-per-day diet, that would be 250 grams.)

In his first edition of *Diet Revolution*, Atkins mentions that Robert Cameron, Blake Donaldson, and John Yudkin took "steps in the right direction," explaining that the flaw in their philosophies was allowing too many carbohydrates, erroneously trying to prevent what he calls the blissful state of "Hey, I'm turning purple every day!" ketosis. He omits any mention of Alfred Pennington or the popular Stillman, whose plan is similar to Atkins's down to the ketosis testing and the "metabolic imbalance" theory that maintains that you'll sneak out extra calories just by breathing and going to the bathroom. He also overlooks *Eat Fat and Grow Slim,* published by British physician Richard Mackarness, MD, in 1958 with a foreword by Mrs. Vilhjalmur Stefansson. It was based on the research done by Stefansson, Donaldson, and Pennington and is so suspiciously like *Diet Revolution* that it's difficult to believe it wasn't its direct inspiration.

13

THE THINKING MAN'S DIET

WALTER KEMPNER, MD, A GERMAN JEW WHO WITH THE HELP OF THE ROCKEFELLER Institute had relocated to the United States to escape Nazi persecution, became a professor at the Duke University School of Medicine in Durham, North Carolina, in 1934. Dr. Kempner had been inspired by the low prevalences of kidney disorders, heart disease, and high blood pressure found in Asia, where a low-protein, low-fat, rice-based diet was a way of life. In 1940 he began testing a specific and very restrictive plan—rice, fruits, sugar, and tea—for patients with these disorders. Renal conditions improved or stabilized, blood pressure dropped, and enlarged hearts became smaller. In 1948, he addressed the New York Heart Association, advocating his diet for the treatment of coronary disease by citing the positive results seen in patients kept on the regimen for as little as 35 days and as long as 3 years. The Rice Diet, as he called it, allowed about 2,000 calories a day, varying somewhat based on the size of the patient. Weight loss was an unavoidable result of the plan, but Kempner thought his diet was too monotonous to be used for that purpose. He also refused to issue a public statement until he had more evidence.

In 1951, Kempner agreed to authorize a Duke University report. It stated that of the 1,800 patients he had treated with rice and fruits, 1,200 showed "marked benefit." The diet, he stated, was very unpleasant and the treatment was tedious and slow, requiring self-discipline and patience. He also believed the diet should be followed only under strict medical supervision.

HE ATE TO LIVE

Nathan Pritikin was an independently wealthy college dropout and inventor who held 50 patents for devices in the fields of electronics, chemistry, and physics. After being diagnosed with "incurable" coronary disease, he researched the literature and discovered Walter Kempner's Rice Diet, in which more than 80 percent of the calories came from carbohydrates. An intense and measured man, Pritikin tested variations of these ideas on his family and himself, changing their diet to one of unprocessed grains, fresh vegetables, fruits, and fish. This was in 1958, when most of America was eating TV dinners, steak, and fast food. "Needless to say," his son Robert was to write about his childhood, "everyone I knew thought we were strange, and, frankly, so did I."

A few years after his heart condition appeared to have been completely reversed, Pritikin became a full-time health reformer, writer, and researcher, in spite of the medical community dismissing the theories and evangelical zeal of an outsider. In 1974 he cowrote what would be the first of several best-selling books, *Live Longer Now*, and began to gain support for his prescription of a low-fat diet and exercise, as opposed to medication and surgery, as treatment for heart disease patients as well as the key to long life. In 1976, the Pritikin Longevity Institute opened for business in a small motel on the beach in Santa Barbara, California. It was literally a last resort—the place where one could go to avert the far more expensive—and at the time very dangerous—coronary bypass surgery. It became so successful that in 1979, the institute relocated to a 125-room hotel in Santa Monica, California, opened a second branch in Florida, and began plans to establish six more facilities in the New York City area. Like the San, John Harvey Kellogg's 19th-century weight-loss facility in Battle Creek, Michigan, it was rapidly transformed from a place where sick people went to get well to a place where healthy and often wealthy people went to lose weight.

EAT THIS, NOT FAT!

Pritikin credited Kempner for his influence in the opening pages of *The Pritikin Permanent Weight-Loss Manual*. Published in 1981, the book's jacket referred to Pritikin as "The Man Who Revolutionized America's Eating Habits" and to his method as "The Safest, Most Efficient Weight-Loss Diet Ever!"

The diet is plant based and thus high in good-quality carbohydrates and low in protein. The foods he recommended eating are, in the following order:

- Vegetables (because they are lowest in caloric density and have high amounts of fiber, vitamins, minerals, and water)
- Fruits (which have more calories because of their sugar content)
- Whole grains (which have less water and more fat, and therefore more calories)

Pritikin also reminded readers that corn, rice, and wheat are *just plants*, a fact that people in their war against carbohydrates often forget.

Pritikin said that the difference between his plan and Kempner's was that on his, you were never hungry. His was also a less monotonous and more nutritionally balanced approach. Meals were broken down into as many as eight "food encounters" a day—brief encounters being preferable. Reminiscent of the San's restrictions, no salt, coffee, or tea was allowed. The only sugar came from fruits. But Pritikin wasn't as strict as predecessors such as Kellogg when it came to meat and alcohol—4 ounces of lean meat or fish were allowed daily, and so was a small glass of wine. Pritikin advocated that his plan was not a diet, but a way of life.

This was also known as the 80-10-10 program, because it was made up of 80 percent complex carbohydrates, 10 percent protein, and 10 percent fat (and thus was considerably lower in fat than the diet recommended by the American Heart Association at the time, which was 50 to 60 percent complex carbohydrates, 10 to 20 percent protein, and 30 percent fat). In 1980, Pritikin partnered with Ted Barash, the advertising executive who made Weight Watchers a household name. Barash was energized by polls indicating that 19 percent of all adult Americans recognized the name Pritikin, and he created a series of seminars. For only $295, people could learn the Pritikin way of diet, health, and life. The goal was to reach $30 million in revenue from these classes by 1982 and then to layer on multiple Pritikin product extensions like spas, cruises, a line of foods, restaurants, and publications. Pritikin, the charismatic inventor, was clearly happy to profit as much as possible from his program, but indicated that a great deal of the proceeds would help fund his research.

Proof that his methods were scientifically sound would have helped him in the Atkins versus Pritikin debates, which began in 1979. "The Fat Feud! Diet Docs Sizzle While Tomes Earn" was the headline on Lynn Darling's piece in the *Washington Post*. While appearing on a Los Angeles television show, "Doc" Pritikin, as he was frequently referred to in the press, adamantly charged that the Atkins diet could result in heart disease, cancer, constipation, and bad breath. Atkins, who sued Pritikin for libel, slander, and $5 million, countered that "Pritikin" was so boring no one would ever stay on it, so it couldn't possibly work and there was no point in even discussing it. "Look at our 500 recipes," argued Pritikin, "soufflés, stir-fried steak, peppers, lemon cheese cake." "Who needs recipes?" countered Atkins, who seemed to imagine that his demographic was made up only of affluent followers. "Just go to a good restaurant and order brisket or lobster with melted butter." And so the high-level medical discussions continued, with Atkins commenting that the only longevity Pritikin was interested in was the longevity of his longevity centers and Pritikin saying that if the high-fat method was so sound, why did he look so much better than his adversary even though he was 63 and Atkins was only 49? "Basically," said an executive at Los Angeles's *Tomorrow Show*, "they both made each other look like asses."

In the 1980s, as the obesity epidemic was beginning to live up to the press notices released in the preceding 30 years, many people tried "Pritikin" for at least a short time, possibly after they gave up on "Atkins." Although sensible and likely to do little harm, it was just as boring as Atkins said it was, stir-fried steak notwithstanding. That reasonable and happy medium—a diet of whole foods, deliciously prepared, a little bit of sugar and fat included—wasn't anywhere on the bestseller lists.

After numerous articles were written about Pritikin's successful reversal of coronary disease with diet and exercise, his company's longevity centers were deluged with phone calls. Death had vindicated Nathan Pritikin, and in spite of the fact that some experts considered the diet too stringent to be effective and perhaps even dangerous, there was no denying that he had mended his own broken heart.

But he was still dead. Many looked at it that way—you can follow the healthiest and most boring diet in the world, exercise, and still not be around to celebrate your 70th birthday. One of the difficulties in convincing people to make dietary changes is that there are no guarantees in life, and eating better and exercising may prevent or even cure a lot of things, but not all of them. And so, in 1980s America, when Pritikin recommended a diet of 10 percent fat, 80 percent complex carbohydrates, and 10 percent protein, the actual eating pattern of America looked more like this: 43 percent fat, 20 percent complex carbohydrates, 20 percent simple carbohydrates (sugar), and 17 percent protein.

America was miles away from Pritikin's ideal, and we were driving in the wrong direction, albeit still moving slowly. In 1961, when 13 percent of the American adult population was labeled obese and 2 years after the Metropolitan Life desirable weight charts were revised to recommend that we weigh less, American men, on average, weighed no more than 2 to 5 pounds more than they had in 1927, and women, on average, weighed 2 to 6 pounds less. "Perhaps they've responded better than men to fat-control campaigns," the *New York Times* theorized in reporting this news. In 1980, 5 years prior to Pritikin's death, the rate had increased slightly. At this point in time, 15 percent of the American adult population was classified as obese.

Nor was anyone suggesting that maybe both fat *and* sugar were the problem, and that you didn't have to pick your poison by choosing between them, you just needed to reduce your intake of both.

It was widely known that the serious case of heart disease from which Nathan Pritikin had suffered prompted his interest in diet and exercise. But there was another reason that he devoted his life's work to the study of energy and the human body, using himself as the primary subject. Pritikin had a rare type of leukemia that had been in remission for many years—a condition kept secret from the public.

The cancer returned in late 1984, and on February 11, 1985, he checked himself into the Albany Medical Center in upstate New York under the pseudonym Howard Malmuth. He had accumulated a complete set of medical records under that name over the previous 20 years; only his family and personal physician knew his real identity at the facility. He was in what must have been devastating pain from treatment for an illness that was now considered terminal, and he spent whatever time he could doing medical research. To that end, he asked a nurse if he could have a razor blade to neatly cut out some relevant articles for his extensive medical files. She didn't have one, but after receiving permission from Pritikin's wife, she gave him a scalpel instead.

Pritikin had requested an hour of solitude every evening between 7:00 and 8:00 p.m., and it was during that time on February 21 that he slashed his wrists. He was pronounced dead at 8:35 p.m. Months earlier, he had requested that upon his death an autopsy be performed, with the results published in the *New England Journal of Medicine* as proof of the efficacy of his diet. The autopsy showed absolutely no remaining evidence of heart disease. The medical report also stated that his arteries were soft, pliable, and disease free—an extraordinary condition in a 69-year-old American male.

Senator George McGovern, who had spent time at the Pritikin Longevity Institute in Santa Barbara and was Pritikin's friend and admirer, gave the eulogy. "The same Nathan Pritikin who took charge of his life 30 years ago when he believed that life was possible, also took charge of his death when he believed life was impossible. I do not mourn his decision," he said.

14

AMERICA, WE HAVE A SITUATION

CERTAINLY, SOME AMERICANS WERE OVERWEIGHT OR OBESE (NOTE THAT THESE classifications are different), although from the 1930s until the late 1970s that *combined* figure hovered at about 25 percent of the population. Then it began a steady rise with each passing year.

The obesity epidemic in America was the unintended consequence of capitalism, science, medicine, and technology colliding. We began to move our bodies less and therefore burn fewer calories at the turn of the century, when automobiles replaced walking and riding bicycles, machines replaced human laborers, large refrigerators and freezers replaced daily trips to the market and kept a huge supply of calories on hand at all times, and rural workers migrated to the city, trading active work for desk jobs. By midcentury, television was not only further encouraging America's sedentary lifestyle, it also introduced us to celebrity diet doctors like Robert Atkins. The most interesting and telegenic doctors became stars, although they weren't necessarily the wisest or most dedicated to the public's best interest.

After Nathan Pritikin's death, Dean Ornish, MD, joined Atkins in heated carbohydrate-versus-fat debates. Ornish, a physician and medical researcher who correctly believed that most of these diets weren't working, somehow thought that he could convince people to follow a plant-based, very-low-fat, very-low-protein, primarily vegetarian diet because that would allow them to eat all they wanted while still losing

135

or maintaining their weight. He ignored the obvious fact that most people had absolutely no desire to live that way.

All foods contain one or more of the following macronutrients: carbohydrates, protein, and fat. These are the basic elements of our diet, and they are what humans have eaten, in varying combinations, throughout time. The ongoing diet debates typically vilified—at times arbitrarily—one particular macronutrient, and the "bad" one kept shifting. The result was a wholesale lack of understanding about what to eat. Potential harm seemed present in every choice, and unlike cigarettes, quitting was not an option. If carbohydrates, fat, and protein were "unhealthy," if fat didn't make you fat, if too much fiber was dangerous and so was too little, and if whole grains, fruits, and vegetables would make you gain weight . . . what *should* you eat? In the face of so much conflicting information and contradictory medical opinions, many Americans seemed to simply throw in the towel.

FOOD FIGHTS

By 1973, Americans had grown accustomed to the low cost and abundance of food—which posed a problem for President Richard Nixon. Americans were spending 15.7 percent of their disposable income on food, less than they ever had before, and less than any other industrialized country. In the same year, Germans spent 22.5 percent of their household income on food, Italians spent 31.9 percent, and the Japanese spent 33.2 percent. But US food prices were predicted to soar. On January 3, the *Wall Street Journal* ran the front-page headline "FATTER FOOD BILLS," warning that a poor fall harvest coupled with increased demand had escalated corn and soybean prices. These were the two main dietary components of the nation's livestock—cows and chickens alike were being fed corn and soybean meal. Since livestock feed accounted for as much as 80 percent of the cost of beef, chicken, and eggs, higher corn and soy prices would translate into higher grocery bills for American families. The price of milk had already increased by as much as 5 cents per gallon, and over the previous 3 months, the cost of eggs had jumped by 20 cents per dozen. An enraged middle class voiced its discontent; housewives organized boycotts and protests, prompting *Time* magazine to label the movement Housewives' Lib. Although some people still remembered World War II rationing and had even lived through the dire circumstances of the Great Depression, for much of the middle class a food shortage or increased food prices was incomprehensible. Agricultural economist Lester R. Brown, head of the Overseas Development Council (and founder of the Worldwatch Institute in 1974), warned that there was a risk of empty meat counters in the months ahead and rationing would be likely. "Americans are sharing food scarcity with Russia," he stated in a 1973 *Newsweek* interview.

The price of sugar was actually going down, but the USDA reacted to demands from the sugar lobby and reduced import quotas for the second time in months—seemingly stabilizing sugar as a commodity. In reality the price would have declined much further if less expensive imports weren't kept out of the American market. The price of everything else— meat, poultry, eggs, fruits, and vegetables—was soaring. The *New York Times* published a question-and-answer session with government, industry, and consumer authorities in an attempt to determine how this could have happened to the best-fed country on Earth and what could be done about it. The leaders criticized Nixon for paying farmers to let some of their fields lay fallow, which now seemed absurd with all of the current shortages. This policy of payment for *not* planting more crops had been enacted about a year earlier, when Nixon was attempting to win the farm vote and further secure his landslide 1972 reelection. Known as the "set-aside" program, it was a subsidy designed to increase the price of basic commodities by keeping land out of production, and it worked—in 1 year US food production dropped more than 2 percent while subsidies to farmers increased by $1 billion. The plan backfired in 1973 when a corn blight occurred, driving prices sky high. This was compounded when Russia bought $1.2 billion of American wheat to make up for its own bad growing season. In addition, the subsidies were mainly issued to large-scale producers and therefore strengthened only the largest corporate farm conglomerates, leaving the remainder of the nation's 2.6 million small farms struggling. The small farmers argued that they were being victimized as the one and only group to fight inflation.

Earl Butz, Nixon's secretary of agriculture, referred to derisively as the secretary of agribusiness, was a former board member of Ralston Purina (animal feed), Stokely-Van Camp (canned goods), and International Minerals and Chemical (fertilizer). It seemed clear that his loyalties lay with corporate farming. To make matters even worse, the government offered the public few helpful suggestions for dealing with this crisis, except for unwelcome ideas like eating less, switching from beef to fish, and skipping expensive snacks and the convenience foods Butz referred to as "built-in maid service." Processed, sweetened snacks and soft drinks had become beloved staples of many Americans' diets, and frozen foods and TV dinners were welcome treats for the millions of American women now working outside the home. Suffice it to say that the Nixon administration's suggestions were not what most Americans wanted to hear.

By September 1974, sugar prices were so high that Hawaiian plantation owners were paying laborers a previously unthinkable $3.20 an hour to hand-harvest the stalks. The US price of raw sugar rose to $33\frac{1}{2}$ cents a pound—more than three times its price just a year earlier. At A&P, a New York City supermarket chain, a 5-pound bag of sugar that had cost 82 cents a year before now cost $2.15. The prices of sweet treats such as baked goods, candies, and soft drinks rose in response. Amazingly, white table sugar had become such an integral part of the national diet that sales remained relatively stable even at the wildly inflated price. Sugar consumption dropped by only 3 percent.

President Nixon instructed Butz, who applauded the high commodity prices that benefited the food industry, to bring prices down fast. Of course, the cost of food turned out to be inconsequential in Nixon's political legacy, but neither man could have known that at the time. Three years after Nixon's resignation, Earl Butz was also forced to resign when he was overheard telling a racially charged joke.

HOW SWEET AND CHEAP IT IS

In the late 1960s, Japanese scientists invented technology that could convert cornstarch into fructose and blend it with glucose. As the name implies, this is the formula for high-fructose corn syrup (HFCS), a sweetener considerably cheaper than cane or beet sugar. It is also at least twice as sweet, depending on the ratio of fructose in the blend.

It is likely that food processors hoping to increase profit margins and decrease costs of goods would have eventually experimented with HFCS. However, escalating sugar prices now coincided with a huge amount of available corn. After Nixon was criticized for the "set-aside" program that subsidized uncultivated land, Butz instructed farmers to plant *all* of their acres "from fencerow to fencerow" with corn and soybeans, initially with the intention of selling it all to the Soviet Union. It was this overproduction of corn that created the surplus that enabled the transition to HFCS to happen almost immediately, and in September 1973, food processing company A. E. Staley took the initiative by expanding its corn processing capacity and increasing production of HFCS at one of its plants by 50 percent.

The incredible thing about HFCS was that it wasn't *just* sweet and cheap, it also extended shelf life and improved product appearance. Beverage manufacturers like Canada Dry and Royal Crown Cola began tinkering with their recipes. Even Coca-Cola gave permission to substitute HFCS for 25 percent of the sugar in its noncola drinks like Sprite and Fanta. Candy manufacturer Hershey Foods Corporation announced that it was strongly considering using HFCS. However, PepsiCo spokespeople said that the company was concerned that fructose changed the taste of cola beverages, so Pepsi would not alter its original formula.

THE CORN RUSH

The floodgates had been opened. Soon industrial food processor Amstar committed to a $20 million expansion of its HFCS capacity. Standard Brands, saying that its HFCS production was sold out until 1976, announced plans for a new $60 million HFCS processing facility in October. American Maize-Products Company, in a joint venture with Cargill, followed suit. Processing high-fructose corn syrup—a business that hadn't existed a few years earlier—was now a booming enterprise. More than 1 billion pounds of the sweet syrup were estimated to sell in

1974, and demand was far outpacing supply. By the middle of the decade, farmers were planting still *more* corn and profits increased even for small farmers.

Coca-Cola was finally able to get a supply of HFCS adequate to allow changing the Coke formula. In 1980, a Coke contained 50 percent HFCS and 50 percent sugar; in 1984, due to the higher profit margins and, according to focus groups, indistinguishable taste, a soda fountain Coke was sweetened with nothing but HFCS. PepsiCo, unable to compete with Coke's reduced ingredient costs, switched to a 50-50 blend of sugar and HFCS in 1984. By 1990, HFCS had almost entirely replaced all other types of sweeteners in caloric soft drinks manufactured in America.

HFCS originally cost about half the price of sugar, and would cost even less as the years went on, supply increased, and eventually, in the early '80s, overproduction drove prices down even more. "Anyone who uses sugar in his products would be foolish if he were not looking into fructose," said a spokesman for Louis Sherry, an ice cream and jam manufacturer. A vice president of Borden's Ice Cream agreed, stating that the company would use HFCS in all of its products if only they could get enough. As sugar prices declined due to the increased use of HFCS, the Coca-Cola Company announced that it would follow a pattern of flexibility—it might use 100 percent HFCS to sweeten bottles and cans of Coca-Cola and caffeine-free Coca-Cola, or not. The manufacturers of both Coke and Pepsi now said that after extensive testing and market research, the results were in and no one could discern a difference in taste. In 8 years, from 1974 to 1982, the consumption of corn syrup increased from 2 to 26 pounds per person, a number that would increase to $73\frac{1}{2}$ pounds per person by 2000.

HOW SWEET AND CHEAP IT ISN'T

In 1976 French-born Harvard nutritionist Jean Mayer was soon to be named president of Tufts University. Mayer had served as diet and health advisor to presidents Richard Nixon, Gerald Ford, and Jimmy Carter, focusing, in part, on combating obesity, which he referred to as a "disease of civilization." At Harvard, he had spent years researching the negative impact of excessive glucose intake on blood sugar level, weight, and heart disease. Thus, he was eminently qualified to speak about HFCS, and he did, warning that scientists were just beginning to understand the effects of this tremendous and sudden increase of fructose in the American diet. The long chains of glucose molecules in starch from corn and other whole grains (which are the carbohydrates that are termed "complex") break down slowly in the digestive tract, giving the body time to cope with the results, he said, while the sugars found in sucrose (table sugar) are absorbed into the bloodstream more quickly. But fructose is the most rapidly utilized of all, said Mayer, and eating a piece of fruit as part of a healthy diet should in no way be confused with "flooding the body with this simple sugar." We know the harm that comes from eating large amounts of sucrose, he concluded, but we know little about the effects of increased fructose consumption, and we should stop using millions of consumers as guinea pigs until we know more.

Food and fructose processors seemed unconcerned about these warnings, and they marketed HFCS as a "natural" sweetener, based on the reasoning that fructose is found in honey and fruits. HFCS was even showing up in tablet and crystal forms as a new kind of miracle drug, sporting claims that it cured everything from alcoholism to obesity. In 1979, the US Postal Service stopped mail distribution of diet booklets that advertised fast and automatic weight loss with fructose tablets.

Whether consuming huge amounts of HFCS was more or less harmful than similar amounts of sugar was still under debate, but the more immediate threat to the American waistline came from the now incredibly low prices for a wide variety of easily available empty-calorie foods. There are 10 teaspoons of sweetener in 12 ounces of Coke, but the lower cost of ingredients allowed consumers to upsize. The Big Gulp, which convenience store chain 7-Eleven debuted in 1980, was a 32-ounce fountain soda. Eventually, a 64-ounce Double Gulp also became available.

In 1910, when US per capita food consumption began to be monitored, Americans were consuming about 91 pounds of caloric sweeteners per year, or 4 ounces per day. In 1980, with figures corrected for "plate waste," use had increased to 143 pounds per year, or about 6.3 ounces per person per day. (HFCS accounted for virtually all of the increase.) An additional

141

2.3 ounces of sugar can be easy to overlook—it's just a 20-ounce Coke—but it translates into 256 more empty calories daily.

Between 1980 and 2000, an additional 400 calories per day were added to the American diet, and it is a reasonable assumption that some if not most of these calories came from HFCS-sweetened sodas, since that is "the number one food consumed in the American diet." Numerous studies have concluded that the brain does not compensate for soft drinks by sending satiety signals that will cause you to eat less of other foods—calories are simply layered on top of calories. That's why those 2.3 ounces of sugar are such an easy oversight.

TREE LARD

As Greg Critser relates in *Fat Land: How Americans Became the Fattest People in the World,* the food processing technology of the 1970s not only made sweeteners cheap and plentiful, it also enabled palm oil to become a less expensive substitute for oils made from the pricier soybeans, cotton, and corn. Like HFCS, palm oil sounded healthier than it really was. More similar to a saturated fat like butter than to a vegetable oil, it was contemptuously referred to by soybean growers as "tree lard." This was actually an underestimation, because lard is 38 percent saturated fat, while palm oil is 45 percent saturated. However, lard, butter, and beef tallow were synonymous with high cholesterol and heart disease, while oil named after an exotic and elegant tree created, for many, the illusion of health. Jean Mayer, a voice of reason once again, tried to point out that palm oil was extremely saturated and potentially deadly, and you might not even know you were buying it. This was because, he said, regulations allowed manufacturers to put any oil they *might* use on their list of ingredients—a product "*might* contain soybean, corn, cottonseed, or palm oil." The consumer had to guess what the ingredients actually were. However, all things being equal, the manufacturer would most likely choose palm oil because it was more stable and offered a far longer shelf life than any alternative.

The popularity of palm oil also frightened the soybean lobby, which demanded a quota on it. They didn't get a quota, but they did receive government subsidies that led to their producing far less expensive animal feed.

WHERE DID ALL THE FIBER GO?

Sylvester Graham and John Harvey Kellogg were great proponents of high-fiber foods like fruits, vegetables, and whole grains, which were, at the beginning of the 20th century, major components of the American diet. High-fiber foods are filling, nutritious, and low in calories. However, as consumption of cheap, sweet, fatty, and refined foods increased, high-fiber food consumption declined.

In the early 1970s, a study published by English researcher Denis Burkitt, MD, suggested that a high-fiber diet might prevent cancer of the colon, the second most prevalent cancer in America at the time. "The major alteration in diet which has taken place has been the replacement of unrefined carbohydrates such as cereals, maize products and brown bread, in favor of refined carbohydrates, which largely means white flour and sugar," Burkitt said. His research suggested that fiber offered protection against colon cancer, as people who ate fiber-rich diets were at significantly lower risk for developing the disease. Jean Mayer and other researchers concurred, although some pointed out that Burkitt's research subjects also didn't eat the high amounts of meat and fat present in the American diet.

High fiber became a new diet fad, and fiber was sometimes called a vitamin despite the fact that it doesn't supply any nutrients to humans.* Fiber became a star. Bread and cereal manufacturers that typically stripped away most if not all fiber in processing were now adding some back in and touting their products as fiber "fortified." Jane Brody of the *New York Times* reported on a shortage of bran in the United States, cautioning that merely adding some fiber back into our poor diets wasn't going to change the negative effects of too much sugar and fat.

---

* It does supply nutrients to animals with four stomachs, like cows and sheep, who, when allowed to graze, break down fiber from grass and hay into nutritious and digestible food that keeps them healthy and without need for antibiotics, and also supplies humans with vitamins and minerals when their meat is consumed. But in humans, fiber passes through the digestive system unchanged, which is beneficial for other reasons, such as preventing constipation and diverticulitis.

FIBER MYOPTICS

Despite the popularity of fiber, few long-term improvements were really made to the American food supply or diet. For example, although Jean Mayer and other health professionals signed a petition demanding that any children's cereals containing more than 10 percent sugar be marketed as high-calorie snacks rather than breakfast foods, their labeling remained the same. Few consumers seemed to care about the high cost of vegetables when there was so much inexpensive and delicious processed food available. When the prices of meat and sugar were deemed too high, people protested loudly and their elected officials reacted quickly to create a steady supply of cheap, sweet, fatty foods. There was a small group of Americans who were becoming suspicious of the food industry at this time and petitioning for change. Adelle Davis, J. I. Rodale, Rachel Carson, Alice Waters, and others were writing and talking about organic produce, humanely treated livestock, the dangers of pesticides and herbicides, and the business of American farming. But this was a very small group compared to the large numbers of outraged people demanding their cheap meat and sugar.

And that, for so many reasons, is unfortunate. High-fiber foods are bulky and require more chewing, so they take longer to eat and make you feel fuller, and eat less. They are nutritious, low in calories, and may prevent not only gaining weight but also a wide variety of diseases. If the country had switched to a diet rich in fruits, vegetables, and whole grains during the fiber fad of the '70s, the obesity epidemic likely would never have become a reality, years would have been added to many lives, and billions of dollars would have been saved on health care.

But a country in love with fast food turned to fast fiber and bought fiber supplements instead. In 1980, there were more than 700 over-the-counter brands available.

PART FOUR

THE DAWNING OF

THE AGE OF
OBESITY

15

HOW MUCH SHOULD I WEIGH AGAIN?

THE BAR FOR THIN WAS LOWERED IN 1983, WHEN THE METROPOLITAN LIFE WEIGHT charts were adjusted for the first time in 24 years—and this time, the numbers moved upward. Reubin Andres, MD, a professor at Johns Hopkins University and clinical director for the National Institute of Aging, offered statistical proof that "ideal" weights had been underestimated. In a long-term study, he said, men of similar ages at the heavier end of the scale had the lowest mortality rates. In a study of women, the very thinnest and fattest were the two groups with the highest mortality rates; the greatest longevity was found in the midrange. These new insurance charts increased the standard for body weight by 1 to 10 percent based on sex and height. The terms "ideal" and "desirable" were no longer used in reference to this standard, according to a Metropolitan Life spokesman, because they "may be misleading."

Ancel Keys agreed with Andres's findings. The results of his 2-decade-long study of more than 12,000 men in the United States, Japan, and Europe indicated that overweight in and of itself was not a risk factor for mortality and that "the risk of premature death is not a simple direct function of relative body weight." David Levitsky, PhD, a nutritionist from Cornell University, added that only about 50 percent of overweight people would experience negative health effects from their extra pounds, and for those who didn't suffer from obesity-related diseases, losing weight wouldn't necessarily lead to greater longevity.

147

To further complicate matters, the statement that Paul S. Entmacher, MD, chief medical director at Met Life, released with the new charts was so convoluted that decoding it practically required a medical degree. In it, he noted that the charts "do not necessarily indicate weights that will reduce the likelihood of illness, nor are the weights those . . . at which a person looks his best." The upward revision, he explained, just reflected what the millions of insured people with the greatest longevity weighed.

On the same day that the new charts were issued, the American Heart Association strongly advised against them, stating that diabetes, high blood pressure, and heart disease *were* correlated with greater weights. Journalist Jane Brody wisely observed that because smoking had not been taken into account in calculating the new tables, the facts that cigarette smokers tend to both be thinner than nonsmokers and to die at significantly younger ages biased the results in favor of greater weight resulting in longer life. "The bottom line is that thinner is still healthier," Brody concluded.

William Castelli, MD, director of the Framingham Heart Study, which had been tracking the health of 5,200 Framingham, Massachusetts, residents since 1949, reported that 82 percent of the smokers fit into the bottom fifth of the weight range *and* had the highest risk of cancer, whereas a thin nonsmoker had the lowest death rate, as well as the lowest heart attack and stroke rates.

IS OBESITY HAZARDOUS TO YOUR HEALTH?

That was the question asked of Theodore B. VanItallie, MD, then professor of medicine at Columbia University and chief of metabolism and nutrition and codirector of Rockefeller–St. Luke's–Roosevelt Obesity Research Center in New York City. His answer? Yes. VanItallie cited recent statistics that indicated that among many other health problems, overweight Americans between the ages of 20 and 45 were almost six times more likely than those of lower weights to have high blood pressure and four times more likely to have diabetes, as well as having a higher incidence of sudden death. He also highlighted the statistical problem of not taking into account the higher proportion of thinner smokers when extrapolating about weight and mortality.

The same question was asked of Paul Ernsberger, PhD, a postdoctoral fellow in neurobiology at Cornell University Medical School and chairman of the National Association to Aid Fat Americans. His answer was no, citing the work of Reubin Andres and Ancel Keys as support. When it came to pointing out flaws in the data, Ernsberger suggested that it was socioeconomic status that had been overlooked; women of low socioeconomic status had a three times higher mortality rate than women in the middle or higher ranges, no matter what their weight.

It was a surprising statement. Four months earlier, the *Journal of the American Medical Association (JAMA)* had published a paper by four preeminent researchers who had analyzed 25 studies on body weight and longevity. They noted that every study had been affected by at least one of three major biases, including not considering the impact of smoking. "The presence of these biases leads to a systematic underestimate of the impact of obesity on premature mortality" was their conclusion, along with the statement that for minimum mortality, Americans on average should weigh at least 10 percent *less* than they did. The following year, *JAMA* published the results of a study of 597 men and 1,126 women, all nonsmokers, and found that those who weighed the most at ages 55 and 65 had about twice the risk of dying within the next few years compared to those of moderate weight. The most common cause of death was cardiovascular disease, followed by cancer. "What's emerging now is that being obese is a risk factor in its own right," stated Millicent Higgins, MD, coauthor of the study and associate director of epidemiology and biometry at the National Heart, Lung, and Blood Institute. The evidence was mounting and seemed conclusive: Americans, on average, should weigh less, not more.

These findings fueled the food bewilderment epidemic, which paralleled the obesity epidemic. When it came to buying and eating, "the American consumer is schizoid," a market researcher who studied the food industry stated. Who could argue otherwise? The best-credentialed scientists in the land couldn't seem to agree on anything, not even how much people should weigh.

MENU BY COMMITTEE

In 1977, the Senate Select Committee on Nutrition and Human Needs issued a report linking six of the leading causes of death in the United States—heart disease, cancer, cerebrovascular disease, diabetes, arteriosclerosis, and cirrhosis of the liver—to a high-fat diet. The committee recommended that Americans reduce their overall consumption of animal fats, table sugar, and salt, while increasing their consumption of fruits, vegetables, and whole grains. Naturally, this government-issue advice resulted in an uproar from the cattle, sugar, corn, soy, and wheat lobbyists. Small-scale farmers who grew fruits and vegetables had no funding to fight for their cause, and so they had no voice in Washington. In the end, the guidelines became a watered-down and confusing version of what they were originally intended to be. Even the USDA couldn't seem to agree on what diet was best for Americans.

Adding to consumers' concerns were growing questions about the use of pesticides and additives. That "schizoid population" was now reading about toxic mercury and possibly carcinogenic polychlorinated biphenyls (PCBs) polluting lakes and rivers and contaminating drinking water and seafood. PCBs were also discovered in chickens and eggs. Another pesticide, 1,2-dibromo-3-chloropropane (DBCP), made headlines when male workers on banana plantations in Central America charged that its application had made them sterile. Temik, or aldicarb, a pesticide used on potatoes, was suspected of being a carcinogen and soon it, too, was prohibited. A congressional auditing agency conducted a study of supermarket meat and poultry and found that 14 percent contained illegal amounts of chemical residues. The official report stated, "Of the 143 drugs and pesticides the General Accounting Office identified as likely to leave residue in raw poultry and meat, 42 are suspected of causing cancer, 20 of causing birth defects, and six of causing mutations." The 1980 *Dietary Guidelines for Americans*, a joint effort of the USDA, the US Department of Health, Education, and Welfare (now called the Department of Health and Human Services), and lobbyists for various agricultural sectors, was now subjected to serious scrutiny.

16

DIETS ARE LIKE STREETCARS

AT THE BEGINNING OF THE 1980S, THE POPULARITY OF THE DIET-BOOK GENRE WAS AT an all-time high, and with good reason—40 million Americans were now considered overweight. The *New York Times* list of the best-selling nonfiction books in 1981 included ones by Richard Simmons (exercise and low calorie), Robert Atkins (low carb and high fat), Nathan Pritikin (low fat, low simple carb, high complex carb, low protein, and low calorie), Craig Claiborne (low salt, low fat, and low calorie), Jane Fonda (exercise and low calorie), and Herman Tarnower (low carb and low calorie), whose Scarsdale diet lived on after his death, just as Pritikin's and Atkins's plans eventually would. Numerous others also lined bookstore shelves. A few of them even contained invaluable information about what you should eat for the rest of your life so you would never have to diet again.

Most of these diets were just thinly veiled attempts to make the low-carb, low-protein, or low-fat theme more appealing, and although many were unpleasant to follow and dieters inevitably regained the weight when they stopped following them, they weren't particularly harmful in the short term. But as in every era in American weight-loss history, some of them were simply insane. The fact that many of them also became bestsellers at a time when the combined weight of the country was continuing to climb suggests that most Americans truly had no idea how to eat anymore.

Judy Moscovitz's Rice Diet, based on the plan developed by Walter Kempner to help very ill patients lose weight under medical supervision, is one such example. Kempner had no interest in turning his rice diet into a fad, but Moscovitz spread the word for him. She sold everything she owned except her television set and her dog so she could move to Durham, North Carolina, to become a "ricer" at Kempner's Duke University clinic, and then she wrote a book—*The Rice Diet Report*—about her experience that also adapted the diet for home use. It is a stringent plan, and potentially dangerous when undertaken without the medical supervision Kempner so strongly recommended. It became a bestseller in 1986.

But perhaps the most ill-advised diet of the decade was Judy Mazel's Beverly Hills Diet. Condemned by the American Medical Association, medical writers, and nutritionists, it quickly became the best-selling nonfiction book in the country, staying at the top of the *New York Times* list for 30 weeks. This "revolutionary" diet by a formerly overweight, self-proclaimed "nutrition guru" with no credentials of any kind seemed reasonable to millions of people in 1981. "Nothing and everything is fattening" was how Mazel cryptically explained her philosophy, adding the magic words: "*You will never be fat again.*"

Mazel had discovered the secret, she said, and it was something called Conscious Combining—eating foods in specific combinations. Fast-digesting fruit must always be eaten alone (that is, never combined with anything from another food group) because otherwise it would get trapped in the stomach by the slower-digesting food and ferment. Proteins must be consumed only with other proteins and fats; carbohydrates other than fruits should only be eaten with other carbohydrates and fats. Like William Hay, whose Hay Diet had prohibited eating protein and carbohydrates in the same meal, Mazel neglected to mention or was unaware of the fact that most foods already contain a combination of protein, carbohydrates, and fats.

She passed along amazing bits of unsound advice: Raw vegetables are not worth eating because they are low in energy; when meat and potatoes are eaten together, the potatoes ferment and turn into vodka in your stomach; the amount of vitamin C in oranges and grapefruits is wildly "overrated"; salt contains hidden sugar.

152

Her diet permits only pineapples or mangos and a few other fruits that aren't "overrated" for the first 10 days, advising readers that any resulting gastrointestinal problems are a good thing, because they will promote additional weight loss. On day 11, ½ pound of unsweetened bread with 2 tablespoons of butter and three ears of corn are allowed; on day 12, it's pineapple and salad; on day 13, apples and buttered baked potatoes. Only mangos are allowed on day 14. And so it goes until the 19th day of the diet, when a complete protein, either lobster or steak with unsalted butter and nothing else, is dinner. The next day, it's chicken for breakfast, lunch, and dinner. The following week, wine and vodka are added to the mix, which surely is a blessing. (According to Mazel, alcohol shouldn't be combined with protein, but it's fine with fruit. She loves strawberries and champagne.)

Clearly, this is not a diet for life—presumably few people other than the anonymous ABC executive mentioned in the book are willing or able to take a whole watermelon along on transcontinental flights. But Mazel was emphatic that the diet could fit any lifestyle, and was especially good for people who drive a lot (like the residents of Beverly Hills). This isn't only because of the need to transport large melons; cars are good for carrying smaller fruits too. She proudly states that she can peel and eat a mango while driving a standard shift—and wearing a white silk dress—without spilling a single drop. (Food writer Roy de Groot, on the other hand, had said that the only way to eat a mango is in a swimsuit and bent over the kitchen sink.)

Mazel died not in an automobile accident, but of a stroke, at the age of 63.

The Beverly Hills Diet may be a terrible way to lose weight, but is a good example of why fads manage to emerge and thrive. They all contain the same basic ingredients: hyperbole, pandering to hope, warnings to ignore the medical establishment (because it's made up of jealous and narrow-minded people), and punishment for the sin of gluttony. No matter how strange the plan, the dieter experiences immediate success from eating what is essentially an extremely low-calorie starvation diet, resulting in a satisfied consumer who spreads the gospel to book-buying friends and family. If someone famous loses weight on the plan, he or she may endorse it or even talk about it on TV. With enough publicity and word of mouth, the diet becomes a trend. Soon, however, it will seem monotonous and dull and impossible to stick with and the dieter will "cheat," and then "cheat" again. Weight is quickly regained—often more than was lost to begin with—and the guilty, bloated dieter tries another diet, perhaps *The New Beverly Hills Diet: The Latest Weight-Loss Research That Explains a Conscious Food-Combining Program for Lifelong Slimhood,* which was the 1996 reinvention of the classic. Here, Mazel told readers that they could finally go public and conduct their affairs out in the open—their affairs with food, that is. "When food is in my mouth, my heart sings and my soul soars. I can match you food fantasy for food fantasy." Then, consciously combining a little religion with the sex and food, she wrote: "Welcome to the world of the Born-Again Skinny."

FIT FOR LIFE

Judy Mazel's book may have been foolish, but at least she was honest about her lack of credentials. This was not the case with the other best-selling "food combining" diet book of the '80s: *Fit for Life,* written by Harvey Diamond, who has a PhD in "natural hygiene," and his wife Marilyn, a certified "nutrition counselor."

The Diamonds theorized that the body is in a daily "elimination cycle" from 4:00 a.m. until noon—during that time, only fresh fruit can be eaten. After noon, you may consume starch or protein, but never together, because the human stomach is incapable of digesting two food groups at once (of course, even a slice of bread contains protein, a fact that apparently was omitted from Harvey Diamond's doctoral-level nutrition courses).

Harvey's alma mater, the American College of Health Science in Austin, Texas, "the only college in the United States to grant the prestigious Natural Hygiene degree," was actually a purveyor of unaccredited correspondence courses. The state ordered it to remove the word "college" from its name and stop issuing degrees of any kind by the end of the decade. Jane Brody wrote about the place in 1988, using Harvey Diamond as an example of how someone could claim to be a nutritionist and "prove it" by presenting a meaningless diploma. Brody told the story

154

of Sassafras Herbert, a poodle with credentials similar to those of the Diamonds and a professional member of the American Association of Nutrition and Dietary Consultants. Sassafras's owner, a physician frustrated by how easy it was to get credentials as a nutritionist, sent a check for $50 in Sassafras's name and received the certificate in return. The poodle also qualified for inclusion in a national directory of what the association called "a Who's Who in the world of modern nutrition."

The reason that this type of quackery was so prevalent, Brody said, is because most states neither licensed nutritionists nor had any standards for qualifying to practice as one. (There are still states where anyone can legally say he or she is a nutritionist without being certified, and others where the requirements are minimal. This is especially frustrating and insulting to the almost 70,000 members of the American Dietetic Association, a group of licensed professional nutritionists.)

WEIGHT LOSS WITH IMMUNITY

Stuart Berger, MD, who had a degree from Tufts University, claimed that by eliminating cow's milk, eggs, yeast, corn, soy, and sugar from your diet you would rebuild your immune system and increase your sexual energy—proving once again that crazy diet advice could be dispensed by experts as easily as quacks. In his *Wall Street Journal* review of the book, Jean Mayer, president of Tufts University, wrote, "It is my hope that no future graduate of Tufts medical school will exhibit as little knowledge of nutrition as does Dr. Berger in this book." Suffice it to say, his quote wasn't used on the back cover of the paperback edition.

Berger was capitalizing on the nationwide confusion over how to lose weight, and adding the emerging panic over HIV infection and its deleterious effect on the immune system as marketing insurance. This was despicable, and very successful. Berger began to appear on television and radio programs with regularity, becoming a doctor for celebrities and a celebrity himself. He was also investigated by the New York State Department of Health for falsifying records, manipulating data, and suspiciously administering both prescription and illegal drugs. When he died in 1994, the coroner's report listed the cause of death as cocaine overdose and extreme obesity. He was 40 years old and 6 feet 7 inches tall, and weighed 365 pounds. His medical license was about to be revoked.

In 1985, *Dr. Berger's Immune Power Diet* enjoyed a 16-week run at the top of the *New York Times* bestseller list until *Fit for Life* edged it out. The Diamonds stayed at the top of the list for 40 weeks.

Fit for Life's coveted position in the number one spot was eventually replaced by *The Rotation Diet,* a combination high-carbohydrate, *very-low-calorie* diet that allowed women only 600 calories for 3 days and 900 for 4 days during the 1st and 3rd weeks of each "rotation." (Men were allowed to consume slightly more.)

The thing about wacky diet plans, especially in the '80s, was that there was always another one waiting to come along. Senator George McGovern's select-committee investigations of fad diets and the official-sounding 1980 *Dietary Guidelines for Americans* seemed to have had little impact. In 1987, the Health, Weight, and Stress Clinic of John Hopkins University had collected almost 29,000 ways to lose weight, of which the director estimated "about 6% are worth a damn."

YOU REFLECT WHAT YOU EAT

By the close of the decade, 33.3 percent of Americans were classified as overweight or obese, which was interesting because that figure had hovered at about 25 percent for decades. The reasons for the sudden increase were varied and difficult to pin down: the daily consumption of fast foods, the wide availability and variety of processed foods, less exercise. Some experts suggested that an actual change had occurred in our DNA to make us more prone to obesity—but even if that were so, it wouldn't account for the massive shift in just one or two generations. Although the greatest prevalence of overweight individuals was among people just above the poverty line, the middle class was rapidly gaining weight too.

What seemed obvious to many was inexplicable to others, and that was the most serious problem of all. It wasn't just that food tasted good—especially the foods created to be "hyperpalatable," a term coined by former FDA commissioner David Kessler, to define foods processed to contain irresistible combinations of sugar, fat, and salt—it was also that, somehow, a lot of people either weren't making the connection that the foods they ate were making them sick or they were too addicted to stop eating them. Or, perhaps most disturbingly, they just didn't care.

EXERCISE MORE?

In 1986, historian Hillel Schwartz published *Never Satisfied: A Cultural History of Diets, Fantasies, and Fat,* in which he argues that for the last 100 years, the cultural tolerance for excess weight had "grown especially narrow," and that "the hostility towards fat extends far beyond physiology." Schwartz meticulously explored what seems like every weight-loss method ever invented—tobacco cures, soap cures, Turkish baths, massage belts, fasting, bath salts, Weight Watchers, starch blockers, health clubs, diuretics, and more than 100 "reducing aids" ranging from Absorbit, a body paste sold in 1907, to the W. B. Reduso Corset for Large Women, another item from the early 20th century. And then, abruptly, he stopped. Weight-loss plans that were bestsellers at the time of his research—those put forth by gurus such as Atkins, Stillman, Mazel, and Pritikin—receive barely a footnote. Instead, Schwartz chooses to end his book by focusing on another 1980s weight-loss phenomenon: Jane Fonda and her incredibly popular workout tapes and companion books.

Schwartz concludes that Americans are in the process of transitioning from "weight-consciousness" to "shape-consciousness," ignoring wealthy urban women and their wistful imitators, the "social x-rays" of Tom Wolfe's classic novel *Bonfire of the Vanities.* Ivana Trump, for example, told reporters in 1986, "It makes me feel powerful to be hungry."

Fonda, whom Schwartz claims without substantiation had been taking amphetamines and using diuretics since she was an adolescent, recommended following a Pritikin-style diet high in complex carbohydrates and low in animal protein and fat to go along with her exercise plan, which, in reference to her long period of anti–Vietnam War activism, Schwartz labels "the diet of the pre-war Vietnamese peasant." He doesn't leave it at that, adding, "As we despoiled and defoliated Vietnam, so now we had to expiate at home, drinking bottled water and eating low on the food chain."

Moving on to the next topic, Schwartz mentions the emerging fear of anorexia and Met Life's revised weight-loss charts to further his argument that dieting may be on the decline, but he also points out that the American Heart Association and the American Cancer Society do not support the idea that people should weigh more than was previously considered ideal. He could not possibly have known that the 25.4 percent of Americans considered "overweight or obese" in the mid-'80s would become 33 percent by the end of the decade, and then skyrocket to a startling 66 percent by 2008. It does seem evident, however, that in spite of the popularity of Jane Fonda, Richard Simmons, Jack LaLanne, health clubs, exercise tapes, jogging, and all of the workout programs marketed in the 1980s, most people had no idea of how to exercise more—or perhaps they just didn't want to.

By 1985 it was estimated that 25 million people, 90 percent of them female, had tried aerobic dance classes, and in 1986 Americans spent $3 billion on athletic shoes. But feeling the burn, like eating meat without potatoes, starts to lose its luster after a while.

LET'S CHARGE LUNCH!

Something else was changing in the American culture—people who wanted everything instantly could have whatever they wanted. As the nation's weight increased, so did its credit card debt. Cards that enabled users to borrow large sums and pay them off in small, high-interest monthly payments were a fairly new concept, and they flourished in the '80s as the advent of computers enabled credit card companies to analyze data and identify the most attractive customers. Those cardholders, flagged by the industry as "revolvers," carried big balances but also were likely to make their high-interest payments. Revolvers were a credit card company's future—they were sent solicitations for additional cards in the mail every month. Most were baby boomers quickly approaching middle age, which was the largest demographic segment in the nation. The radicals of the 1960s and 1970s had grown up. A lot of marijuana-smoking hippies turned into cocaine-snorting Yuppies during the Ronald Reagan administration, at the same time that the movie-star president and his wife were promising a return to the American dream.

The disappointment of not having it all (for a lot of women "all" now meant a great career, a happy marriage, wonderful children, and plenty of money, whereas for men it meant a great and *highly lucrative* career, a happy marriage, power, and enough free time to spend with their wonderful children) strongly attracted these Yuppies to forms of more immediate gratification: spending too much, trying a new get-thin-quick scheme from one of the 300 available diets books, cracking open a self-help book, or simply taking a pill—anything to help you forget that you weren't achieving perfection the way movie stars Jane Fonda and Ronald Reagan suggested you should. "It's the '80s and I forgot to get rich!" was a popular watercooler joke, usually accompanied by a slap to the side of the head and a grin. Everyone smiled in agreement, because they all knew that although you could never be too thin or too rich, you were unlikely to become either. (However, you could pretend that you were both by having a new procedure called liposuction. In 1986, 100,000 Americans paid $2,000 to $4,000 for the procedure.)

By 2009, credit card defaults totaled more than $75 billion. Although it's true that credit card companies didn't force us to supersize our debts any more than McDonald's forced us to supersize our bodies, they both made it hard to resist. There is mounting evidence that humans are bad decision makers, even when we are given the information we need to make good choices. A 2004 University of Maryland study showed that people who wouldn't be able to pay off their balances within 6 months would still pick a credit card with a "teaser" rate of 4.9 percent for 6 months over one with a teaser rate of 7.9 percent for 12 months, even though the rate after either introductory period would jump to 16 percent, making the first option cost significantly more. Obviously, we have difficulty analyzing the consequences of our actions and let immediate gratification outweigh future pain. It doesn't explain why some people neither spend too much nor weigh too much, but it begins to help us to understand why so many do.

17

HOW MUCH SHOULD I EXERCISE AGAIN?

THE PRESIDENT'S COUNCIL ON PHYSICAL FITNESS AND SPORTS HAS BEEN IN existence since 1956, which means that it predates the equally ineffective war on drugs by more than a decade. Press coverage of the council's recommendations has been intermittent, but its lack of sufficient funding has remained consistent. President Dwight D. Eisenhower, perhaps motivated by worry over his own health after experiencing a massive heart attack, created the council to enhance the health of the nation's children. Shane MacCarthy, Boston resident, County Cork, Ireland, native, and brusque former chief orientation officer for the CIA, was named the first executive director of what was originally called the President's Council on Youth Fitness in October 1956, prompting him to say: "Here in America our pattern of living has become so mechanized and education so crowded that it has pushed physical training into a secondary position." MacCarthy was critical of America's young men, harshly stating that because more than one-third of all potential draftees were being rejected, as a nation, if things didn't improve quickly, we might all "wake up dead." We had endless opportunities *not* to be active, he believed. We no longer walked, we drove, and the new power steering, power brakes, and automatic transmission meant that we were barely moving our arms and legs when we did. To make things worse, a survey of schoolchildren had revealed that 10 percent were overweight or obese. Vice President Richard M. Nixon, who had little interest in sports except as a spectator, was nevertheless named chairman of the committee.

The message of the council was unfocused, and soon the definition of fitness was broadened to include not only physical well-being, but also mental, emotional, social, and spiritual health, as if simply getting in better shape wasn't enough of a goal. There was a hazy agreement that fitness should begin at home and yet involve all facets of the community, and that girls should be given equal attention in the schoolyard.

In 1956, Eisenhower added a citizens' advisory committee to work alongside MacCarthy's council. Its mission was equally broad and difficult to comprehend, let alone achieve: "to alert our community on what can and should be done to reach the much desired goal of a happier, healthier and more totally fit youth in America." Members of the new committee included movie stars Gary Cooper, Bing Crosby, and Esther Williams and television star Arthur Godfrey. After a year, the *New York Times* reported that the council and advisory committee had neither delivered any blueprint for fitness nor even agreed upon a definition of the word. That wasn't surprising, since it had no budget and relied upon meager appropriations from various departments of the president's cabinet; that year the Departments of Labor; Defense; Agriculture; the Interior; and Health, Education, and Welfare contributed a combined total of $143,000. Nixon, who never developed any interest in the project, told MacCarthy not to expect any additional funding, even though he thought that more physical activity might curb the nation's growing problem of juvenile delinquency (which may or may not have been accurate, but surely missed the point).

John Fitzgerald Kennedy is the president who is probably most closely associated with a national physical fitness directive. It was during the short period of his presidency that Americans seemed to become interested in low-cost, all-American physical activities, such as hiking and team sports. Fitness was an important issue for Kennedy. As president-elect he had written an article for *Sports Illustrated* magazine titled "The Soft American," in which he spoke of the "general physical decline of American youth" and outlined his plans to address the problem. He had seen warning signs when so many potential recruits were rejected for the armed services during the Korean War, he said, and he was now seriously alarmed about the laziness of the nation's youth. Two researchers at New York's Columbia–Presbyterian Hospital had recently published the results of a 15-year study of children in America, Austria, Italy, and Switzerland. The children of the United States—the country that was supposed to be the best fed and to have the highest standard of living—performed deplorably. Of the six tests administered to the children to gauge muscular strength and flexibility, 57.9 percent of the American children failed one or more, compared to 8.7 percent of the Europeans. Kennedy said that the "flabbiness" of American youth was "a menace to our security."

Few people of the time were aware that their trim, athletic-looking president actually suffered from debilitating chronic back pain. He was limited in his own physical activities to swimming and sailing. His athleticism was an illusion, but he and his family represented a fantasized version of the American dream—affluent, slim, active, beautiful people playing fiercely competitive touch football together on a Sunday afternoon. Many of the Kennedy family's friends were true athletes—Secretary of the Interior Stewart Udall even climbed Japan's Mount Fuji, a peak that is more than 12,000 feet tall. On the first of what would become the Kennedy administration's famous 50-mile (in 20 hours or less) hikes, Attorney General Bobby Kennedy, walking in oxford shoes and a dress shirt, was said to have finished the race. The hiking craze so captivated the nation that it was necessary for the council to publish a cautionary warning that inactive people should begin with moderation, check with their doctors, and wear proper shoes and socks.

WASHINGTON, D.C.
IMMEDIATE RELEASE
FEBRUARY 12, 1963

The President's Council on Physical Fitness recommends hiking as an excellent activity for improving physical fitness and is pleased to note the current interest in that form of exercise. The Council advises those who have not been exercising regularly to begin moderately and to gradually increase the amount and

162

intensity of the activity. This caution applies to any exercise program including walking and hiking.

Begin by walking a distance—and at a pace—that does not result in undue fatigue. Day by day increase the distance and the vigor. If you have not had a medical checkup recently, talk with your physician before engaging in a rigorous fitness program. Before undertaking long hikes, be sure you are wearing the proper shoes and socks.

A fifty mile hike is a fine challenge for the Marines and other persons who are in good physical condition. The Council is pleased to note the number of people who are sufficiently fit to cover that distance.

The Council also urges all citizens to participate regularly in a planned program of physical activity, consistent with their physical condition, as an essential aspect of a balanced life.

Paul Dudley White, who had gained prominence as President Eisenhower's heart specialist and was frequently interviewed about diet and fitness, said that he was happy people were moving and that their feet would give out long before their hearts did. The country was filled with energy and hope. Walking 50 miles seemed like a wonderful thing to do.

IT'S SUPERMAN!

In this promising new atmosphere, even Superman was summoned to help Americans shape up. A story line planned for a late fall 1963 issue of the comic book, to be issued in cooperation with the fitness council, was to feature President Kennedy asking the Man of Steel for a favor: Would he visit the nation's schools and teach students some new exercises? He would also be asked to skywrite this message along the way: SOUND MINDS IN SOUND BODIES—JOIN THE PRESIDENT'S PHYSICAL FITNESS PROGRAM. That issue, which would have gone on sale in December of 1963, was never published. The original art was given to the president's widow.

AMERICA'S BEST-KEPT SECRET

Vice President Lyndon Baines Johnson completed Kennedy's term and was elected president in 1964. Johnson, you'll recall, had suffered a heart attack and spoke afterward of watching his cholesterol. But he lacked his predecessor's passion for physical fitness. The president's council wasn't dissolved, but no one seemed to be very interested in moving it forward. New York advertising firm Young and Rubicam was hired to boost the council's flagging profile, but its creative efforts were a far cry from Superman: a sad-looking, chubby boy cradled a big jar marked "COOKIES" with one hand and gripped a cookie in the other, and this was accompanied by the headline: "What are you doing about your son's nickname?" The copy continues, "There is no excuse for the overweight, out of shape youngster, boy or girl, and the embarrassing nicknames they go by. What about your school's physical education program? Insist on a daily 15-minute session of honest exercise."

Twenty years later, even those 15 minutes of game time were in peril. When Nixon took office in 1969, he was still disinterested in the President's Council on Physical Fitness and Sports (renamed as such in 1968) and did little more than create a few new executive positions and, once more missing the point, authorizing the publication of a quarterly fitness journal. The council continued to languish under presidents Gerald Ford (1974 to 1977) and Jimmy Carter (1977 to 1981.) With public school budgets stretched tight, by 1987 physical education was mandatory in just 17 states, and only a third of all students had daily gym classes. Forty percent of children between the ages of 5 and 8 were said to have elevated blood pressure, high blood cholesterol levels, and sedentary lifestyles. George Allen, the former pro football coach who was appointed chairman by President Reagan in 1981, called this lack of fitness "the best kept secret in America today." Parents, who might have been working out to fitness tapes (which were, incidentally, one of the main reasons people cited for purchasing videocassette players in the early 1980s), seemed oblivious to all of the little hands in the cookie jar. A 1987 Harris Poll showed that 9 out of 10 parents thought their children were in great shape when in fact, according to a study released by the president's council, 40 percent of

164

school-age boys and 70 percent of school-age girls could do no more than one pullup; 33 percent of the boys and 50 percent of the girls were unable to run a 10-minute mile. Unfortunately, this was the last year for the president's council fitness surveys, which were discontinued due to budgetary pressures. Sadly, the end of collecting these valuable metrics coincided with an era in which the obesity rate of America's youth rose to 27 percent for children ages 6 to 11—a rate nearly triple the 10 percent of children who were considered obese in the 1950s.

FRENCH CHILDREN DON'T GET FAT

In 2004, when an uptick in childhood obesity was reported in France, the government responded swiftly—children between the ages of 5 and 12 were weighed at school and reports containing their weights and body mass indexes were sent to their parents, along with instructions explaining how to interpret the numbers. Parents then attended meetings with local physicians and dietitians about ways to prevent or reverse the trend with diet and exercise, and children were taught about portion control and good nutrition. Vending machines selling sodas and snacks were banned from school campuses and exercise was encouraged. The plan was simple, clear, and effective—the obesity rate declined before stabilizing in 2007.

SEE YOU AT THE GYM! OR NOT: THE PHYSICAL INACTIVITY EPIDEMIC

In 1960, only about 24 percent of adult Americans said that they worked out. By 1981, the year President Reagan took office, that figure had doubled. More Americans than ever before reported engaging in strenuous nonwork-related exercise and endurance sports like running in marathons. Health club memberships were up, as were sales of running shoes and sports equipment. President Reagan, the oldest person ever to be elected president, became actively involved with the fitness movement, and about 50 percent of adult Americans said they were physically active during the 1980s. Perhaps baby boomers, who were now thirtysomethings headed toward middle age, were trying hard to pretend they weren't.

When President George H. W. Bush took office in 1989, he was as disinterested in government intervention in diet and fitness as many of his predecessors had been. After appointing Arnold Schwarzenegger—a former Olympic bodybuilder and movie star who harbored Republican ambitions of his own—as council chairman, he stepped away from further involvement. The exercise trend, referred to by *Time* magazine in 1981 as a "national obsession," suffered a reversal. Most parents became as inactive as their kids, who were not only getting little to no exercise at school, they were no longer walking there either—the percentage of children walking to school decreased by 60 percent between 1977 and 1995. After-school free time was often spent with televisions, computers, and junk food—and junk food commercials. By 1995 American children were exposed to, on average, an astonishing 10,000 food commercials a year—and they weren't being paid for by broccoli farmers. To counter this, the government allocated states an average of $50,000 to teach children to eat right. To put this figure into perspective, Kellogg's was spending $32 million a year to advertise one product—Frosted Flakes.

In 1995, *Time* magazine reported, "The national fitness fixation has come off the hinge." Two years earlier, the President's Council on Physical Fitness and Sports had published the depressing statistics that 25 percent of the adult population was completely sedentary and another 33 percent was barely active, calling it "an epidemic of physical inactivity." It was, indeed, a return to 1960 statistics, but with more food. Sports scientists and epidemiologists believed that the fitness focus had wrongly been placed on performing rigid and regimented exercise routines, which most people disliked, had no time for, and couldn't afford to participate in. The surgeon general's 1996 report joined "physically fit" with "physically *active*," recommending something as simple as walking at a moderate pace on most, if not all, days of the week. But even this didn't happen.

A small segment of the population, primarily but not only the educated, affluent, and urban, maintained reasonable fitness levels, but the majority of people did not, including many from that elite socioeconomic group. It turned out that getting people to exercise was even more difficult than convincing them to eat fewer calories, although the health issues that accompany inactivity are similar to those seen with poor diet, such as diabetes, heart disease, certain cancers, high blood pressure, and osteoporosis. Working out requires time and effort. Eating less is something you can do at home, and you don't even have to buy a new pair of sneakers. Assessments of physical fitness also are not easily quantified. To accurately measure an individual's fitness level, he or she would need to undergo tests for balance, agility, coordination, muscle strength, cardiorespiratory function, flexibility, and body composition. Stepping on a scale is certainly simpler.

HEAVY LIFTING

In 1995 America, every age group was heavier than the comparable group had been 10 years earlier. Sixty-year-olds were heavier; fifty-year-olds were too, and so on down the demographic age scale. Fifty-eight million people now weighed at least 20 percent more than their optimal body weight as determined by their BMI, earning them the designation of "obese." That fewer people were smoking was suggested as one possible reason. Those who quit might gain about 4 to 6 pounds—a better than fair trade for health, experts concluded—but that small increase was hardly enough to cause the extreme jumps in weights that were being seen. It was shocking and also seemed inexplicable to the University of Pennsylvania's Albert Stunkard, MD, founder of the school's Center for Weight and Eating Disorders, who admitted, "All of us were stunned. It runs counter to what we as a nation seem to be doing."

Was it possible that the experts were not only missing the forest for the trees, but also camping out in the wrong woods? Could the scientists, academics, and journalists—who as a group were generally urban, affluent, and educated—be blind to the reality in the rest of the country? Seemingly, this was the case. So many obvious signs seem to have been missed. Stunkard postulated that the fitness movement had been too narrowly focused and had reached mostly the upper and upper-middle classes, missing the rest of the population.

But the upper and upper-middle classes were hardly exempt. Nor were the wealthy. Media sensation Oprah Winfrey, who began yo-yo dieting her way into the new millennium, carried a svelte 123 pounds on her 5-foot-7-inch frame when she was showing off her figure in sexy jeans and boots during sweeps week back in 1987. It was her most-watched episode to date, with 18.4 percent of households with televisions tuning in. Oprah said she got her amazing results with Optifast, a very-low-calorie liquid starvation diet plan. Drinking it, of course, then became a nationwide weight-loss trend. Part of the problem surely was those hundreds of worthless fads that almost always resulted in regaining more weight than you lost, just as if Sisyphus's rock not only rolled back down the hill every time he got it up to the top, it rolled just a little *further* downhill each time. Unrealistically fast, difficult, and unsustainable methods are generally followed by disappointment, and disappointment can easily spawn apathy. Stabilizing the American obesity rate was becoming more illusive by the year.

18

FAT-FREE FAT

ANOTHER EXPLANATION OFFERED FOR THE "SUDDEN" INCREASE IN AMERICA'S WEIGHT was the explosion of packaged, fat-free foods on the shelves of every grocery store in the country. In 1995, more than 1,300 new fat-free or low-fat products were introduced to the marketplace. In the following year, the fat substitute olestra received FDA approval and was used to make many processed foods. People were eating "diet" snack foods with abandon, apparently confusing fat-free with calorie-free and somehow believing that devouring an entire box of cookies made sense. The so-called Snackwell Effect is named for this phenomenon. It describes the irrational behavior that can follow a positive change and sabotage one's efforts, like replacing all of your lightbulbs with energy efficient models and then leaving the lights on all day.

THERE'S NO SUCH THING AS A FAT-FREE LUNCH

Olestra is a compound that is just like oil except for a few key differences: It's indigestible and a laxative; it prevents the fat-soluble vitamins A, D, E, and K from being properly absorbed; and it occasionally causes a problem known as anal leakage. Nevertheless, with this fat-free fat Procter and Gamble had dreamed the impossible dream. The company began petitioning for FDA approval in 1971. Marion Nestle, PhD, in her significant 2002 book *Food Politics,* describes how olestra, unique in being "the first additive likely to be consumed in large quantities," was ultimately given FDA approval as an ingredient in savory snacks (the packaging of which had to display an explicit warning about potential negative side effects) despite the strong objections raised by the Center for Science in the Public Interest about both physiological issues and scanty research. Nestle singles out olestra as "the most ironic of techno-foods; . . . designed to encourage people to eat more top-of-the-*Pyramid* snack foods." These new salty snacks would become perfect candidates for the Snackwell Effect.*

Olestra became an ingredient in a variety of chips and crackers. It had cost Procter and Gamble an estimated $500 million for research, patent extension, campaign contributions, lobbying, and, finally, marketing. It was given the brand name of Olean and promoted as the "healthy," soy-based fat-free frying oil after exclusive rights for its use were sold to Frito-Lay, a division of PepsiCo. In 2003, the FDA said the label warning consumers of olestra's presence in a product no longer was required, meaning that packages of fat-free Pringles, Lay's Light, and Ruffles Light potato chips, as well as many other snacks, mentioned it only in the ingredients list.

Olestra turned out to be a gamble that never paid off for P&G. The negative press along with all of the uncomfortable gastrointestinal side effects prevented it from becoming the multibillion-dollar earner they had projected, although in 1998 P&G estimated that Americans had consumed 28 million snacks fried in Olean and had therefore "saved" 2 billion calories. Nevertheless, those figures were 30 to 40 percent below production estimates. P&G decided to temporarily put aside plans for seeking FDA approval for broader usage of Olean in food items like cookies and french fries.

But the problem with this synthetic fat was not only its image. The initial FDA approval had taken decades, and in the meantime, most Americans had wearied of making fat the enemy and gone back to vilifying carbohydrates.

---

* Snackwells, to be clear, have no olestra. Each Devil's Food Fat Free 50-calorie cookie contains sugar, enriched flour (wheat flour, niacin, reduced iron, thiamine mononitrate [vitamin B$_1$], riboflavin [vitamin B$_2$], folic acid), high-fructose corn syrup, corn syrup, fat-free milk, cocoa (processed with alkali), glycerin, emulsifiers (soy lecithin, mono- and diglycerides), leavening (baking soda, sodium aluminum phosphate, calcium phosphate), gelatin, cornstarch, modified corn starch, chocolate, salt, potassium sorbate added to preserve freshness, and artificial flavor.

RETURN OF THE KILLER CARBS

With a pent-up demand for real (not chemical) fats, America went into a fat-eating frenzy, and carbohydrates returned as public enemy number one. By the end of the 1990s, the top four spots on the *New York Times* paperback nonfiction bestseller list were low-carb plans, including *Dr. Atkins' New Diet Revolution* ("new" because he said so, not because of any major changes), *The Carbohydrate Addict's Diet, Suzanne Somers' Get Skinny on Fabulous Food, and Sugar Busters!* The latter was the joint effort of a cardiovascular surgeon, an endocrinologist, a gastroenterologist, and the CEO of a Fortune 500 company who trademarked their catchy title. The message of *Sugar Busters!* is simple: *"Sugar is toxic!"* The authors prescribe a low-carbohydrate, low-fat, low-calorie diet that contains vegetables, some fruits, whole grains, and lean meats.

When it was unthinkable to go another day without potatoes or pasta, the other end of the spectrum was still available—physician Dean Ornish's *Eat More, Weigh Less,* a well-documented, spiritual approach to a very-low-fat, high-complex-carbohydrate, high-fiber, low-calorie diet that was as boring and difficult to stay with as Nathan Pritikin's had been. To Ornish's credit, he includes recipes from some of the most famous chefs of the time, including Wolfgang Puck and Deborah Madison. The ingredients list for Cheese Blintzes with Fresh Fruit, a noble effort by Myrna Melling, includes oil-free egg substitute, fat-free milk, vegetable oil spray, fat-free cottage cheese, and 2 teaspoons of sugar along with the fruit. There were many other, less successful "new and revolutionary" ways to lose weight, but since there are only three macronutrients and you can only count grams of each or, more realistically, count calories, there are only so many possible permutations and combinations. All of the plans ultimately wind up as remembrances of things past without the pleasure of *la petite Madeleine.*

19

THE PILL ON THE
COVER OF *TIME*

IN APRIL OF 1996, THE FDA APPROVED THE DIET DRUG REDUX, AN APPROPRIATELY named pill in an industry where everything old is new again. Redux, as marketer Wyeth-Ayerst Laboratories spun it, was a drug for the morbidly obese and should be used only for a short period of time. Instead, 3 months after approval, 85,000 prescriptions were being written every week and the national weight-loss companies Nutrisystem and Jenny Craig were recommending it to their customers. *The Redux Revolution,* by Sheldon Levine, MD, said it was "the most important weight-loss discovery of the century." In September, *Time* put the drug on its cover, calling it the "Hot New Diet Pill."

Wyeth-Ayerst Laboratories, at the time a division of American Home Products, was said to have projected a sales goal for Redux of $1 billion over a period of 5 years and spoke of rarified plans to "educate" the public about obesity (as opposed to simply hawking the pill to every doctor in town). They already had salespeople speaking with thousands of general practitioners around the country, convincing them that a safe and effective prescription for weight loss was, at long last, a reality. An analyst for Montgomery Securities in San Francisco called it "probably the fastest launch of any drug in the history of the pharmaceutical industry."

Redux was also well named because its active ingredient was dexfenfluramine, a refined version of fenfluramine, the compound that put the "fen" in "fen-phen," the two-pill diet drug cocktail that had become a pharmaceutical bonanza a few years earlier. Research on fenfluramine and appetite control had begun decades earlier, when MIT neurologist Richard Wurtman, MD, and his nutritionist wife Judith Wurtman, PhD, were researching a connection between the hormone serotonin and appetite. They theorized that some people might be unknowingly self-medicating for depression by eating high-carbohydrate diets, because carbohydrates increase the level of the hormone serotonin in the brain. Serotonin, they knew, creates a sense of well-being and, they speculated, satiety. Fenfluramine is a selective serotonin reuptake inhibitor, or SSRI. SSRIs block the brain's reabsorption of serotonin, making it more available in the brain's synapses. In 1987, Prozac (fluoxetine) became the first SSRI to be successfully marketed as an antidepressant. Eli Lilly, the pharmaceutical giant that introduced it, considered also marketing fluoxetine as an antiobesity drug and reported that it was conducting clinical trials to that end in 1986. They discontinued the plan when they couldn't overcome the problem of fatigue. In the early 1970s, a fenfluramine compound called Pondimin had been introduced as a miracle diet pill, but it had failed for the same reason.

THE UPS AND DOWNS OF DIET PILLS

Fenfluramine as an antiobesity remedy languished for years, because although it was an effective appetite suppressant, it also tended to make people fall asleep. In the early 1980s, however, a researcher combined fenfluramine with the amphetamine-like phentermine, and this solved the fatigue problem—the phentermine woke you right back up. You were, in effect, taking an "upper" and a "downer" together, not unlike the Benzedrine combinations prescribed in earlier decades. After a 4-year study of 121 subjects, who had an average weight loss of 32 pounds, the results were released and the craze began. Since both halves of the fen-phen recipe already had FDA approval, doctors simply tore two prescription forms from their pads and instructed patients to use both in an "off-label" use (one for which the drug—or drugs, as in this case—is not approved by the FDA). With its patent on fenfluramine soon to expire,

Wyeth-Ayerst Laboratories (which did not make phentermine) obtained FDA approval for dexfenfluramine, a new drug related to fenfluramine that usually would not cause fatigue. That was the new miracle drug they called Redux, and in 1996 it had a marketing budget of $52 million just for its initial launch.

The side effects for Redux and fen-phen were similar. Some were mild, including dry mouth, diarrhea, and loss of libido, but others were potentially dangerous. Laboratory animals had suffered brain damage while on the drugs, but the FDA's major concern was the possibility of a fatal disorder called primary pulmonary hypertension, a disease that damages the heart valves and arteries in the lungs. These risks were weighed against the rewards of decreased obesity and thus reduced heart disease, cancer, and diabetes. The drug was approved.

When it delivered $300 million in sales in 1996, Redux appeared to be everything Wyeth-Ayerst had hoped for, but the good news didn't last. In July 1997, 24 previously healthy women who had taken either fen-phen or Redux were diagnosed with a rare heart ailment, and then 9 additional women developed similar problems. Jenny Craig immediately stopped recommending the drug to clients. Nutrisystem did as well, and also began to suggest taking a product that contained the herbal weight-loss remedy ephedrine instead. In September 1997, at the FDA's request, Wyeth-Ayerst voluntarily recalled both Redux and fenfluramine. Almost 21 million prescriptions had been written for the two drugs during 1996.

It was estimated that there had been almost 6 million users prior to the recall. Redux ultimately cost Wyeth more than $21 billion in legal fees and settlements, and the new millennium began with the FDA being very cautious about approving prescription antiobesity pills. That caution, in turn, increased the demand for over-the-counter diet products.

FAT BURNERS AND STARCH BLOCKERS

The Dietary Supplement Health and Education Act of 1994 (DSHEA, pronounced D'Shay) had taken authority over dietary supplements away from the FDA (which had previously regulated them in the same way as conventional foods), and now the manufacturers of vitamins and weight-loss products were no longer under its control. Marion Nestle refers to this as "the industry's crowning achievement," because it allowed manufacturers to make efficacy claims without having the support of scientific evidence as long as they were properly worded, and also because they no longer had to prove their products were safe before putting them on the market. Instead, the FDA had to prove a product *unsafe* if it wanted to recall it. In terms of diet aids, this legislative change brought a return to the days of quack remedies like Allan's Anti-Fat, the 1878 "remedy for corpulence." Allan's Anti-Fat contained bladder wrack (also referred to as fucoxanthin), a seaweed that was the original source of supplemental iodine. The remedy contained so much fucoxanthin that it induced hyperthyroidism. It is currently an ingredient in a variety of weight-loss products, including Apidexin, which its manufacturer calls "the world's strongest fat burner."

The most popular supplements in the mid-1990s were those referred to as herbal fen-phen in homage to and memory of the real thing. The herb in these products was ephedra, which was harvested from shrubs grown in Asia. Ephedra (also referred to as ma huang or ephedrine) had been used in Chinese medicine for thousands of years and in American cold remedies since at least the 1920s. For mental stimulation and weight loss, it was thought to be even more effective than Benzedrine, the diet pill that first entered the market as a less expensive alternative to ephedrine. It was also an ingredient in methamphetamine. At correct dosages, it worked as a diet aid because it had amphetamine-like effects on the body; it was, essentially, a shot of speed. By 1999, it was being used in more than 200 diet pills, powders, drinks, and bars.

One of the most widely consumed of these products was Metabolife 356. Michael Ellis, a former police officer and the CEO of Metabolife International, knew a lot about this particular herbal remedy. Eleven years earlier, he and his childhood friend Michael Blevins had been arrested following an FBI raid on Blevins's house in Rancho Santa Fe, California, that revealed a methamphetamine lab and enough chemicals to produce 50 pounds of the highly addictive illegal street drug. In 1989, Ellis pleaded guilty to a reduced charge of facilitating a drug deal

175

and received 5 years of probation. Blevins did the time. Following his parole, he and Ellis formed Metabolife. Legally compounding ephedrine proved lucrative; Metabolife 356 had a sales projection of $900 million in 1999. The FDA questioned Ellis about possible deleterious side effects caused by the supplement. He responded that Metabolife 356 was "claims free."

Herbal supplements—which are not regulated by the FDA—aren't necessarily manufactured under standardized conditions and often don't contain the amount of the herb (or anything else) that appears on the label. Taking less of the recommended dose may be ineffective, and taking more may be dangerous or even lethal. In addition, while a particular herb may be safe on its own, when combined with caffeine or other herbs it may be hazardous. But these interactions are rarely tested, as there is no profit in disproving a product's safety. As early as 1993, physicians began to submit hundreds of negative reports to the FDA—including documented deaths—that seemed to implicate ephedrine diet supplements.

In 2003, Steven Bechler, an overweight 23-year-old rookie with the Baltimore Orioles, was trying to lose 10 to 15 pounds fast. To that end, during spring training on February 17th, he was wearing more than one layer of clothes in the 85°F heat, had eaten very little or not at all, and was taking Xenadrine RFA-1, an ephedra-based dietary supplement. When he collapsed and died, his body temperature was 108°F.

In less than 2 years, between 2002 and 2004, ephedra was linked to 10 deaths, 13 cases of permanent disability, and more than 60 other serious adverse effects, but it was the death of a professional athlete that brought the dangers of the supplement into the national spotlight. The FDA banned weight-loss supplements containing ephedra in 2004, following congressional hearings. Ellis, as it turned out, had lied to the FDA about his products being claims free. Metabolife had received more than 13,000 customer complaints dating back to 1997. In 2008, Ellis pleaded guilty to making a false statement to the FDA and was sentenced to 6 months in federal prison and fined $20,000. But Ellis wasn't the only villain. Numerous other manufacturers had lied, and there also was evidence that safety reports had been falsified.

DIET PILLS ARE LIKE STREETCARS, TOO

Hydroxycut was another of the best-selling diet-aid brands in the country. Made with green tea extract, it quickly replaced ephedra as the hot new diet supplement. Along with the tea extract, which is yet another substance that speeds up metabolism, the product's list of ingredients included oolong and white teas, caffeine, fruit extracts, and herbs. In May 2009, a 20-year-old previously healthy man died from liver failure after using Hydroxycut. In all, 23 cases of serious liver conditions were reported, as were muscle damage that could lead to kidney failure and heart problems. Nine million units had been sold in 2008. The FDA requested an immediate recall of Hydroxycut following the young man's death, and Canadian manufacturer Iovate Health Sciences and its American distributor voluntarily complied.

After the Hydroxycut incident, many people (including television pundits) expressed shock and dismay that our FDA hadn't done a better job of protecting the public from dangerous supplements. They clearly were unaware that supplements are innocent until proven guilty and the agency had little power over them unless they could prove substantial harm, by which time it was too late. An article in the *New York Times* about the Hydroxycut recall asked whether the FDA had "adequate authority to regulate the dietary supplement industry and provide consumer protection." The answer was obvious, but a country both at war and going through the worst economic time since the Great Depression quickly refocused on other priorities.

Synephrine, which is usually referred to as bitter orange, replaced ephedrine in numerous supplements following the 2004 ban, including the "fat burners" Stacker 2 and Stacker 3. Although not considered as effective as ephedrine, synephrine raises metabolism when taken at high doses along with caffeine. In 2009, supplements containing acai berry and Iovate Health Sciences' *Hoodia gordonii,* which is a succulent plant, were being heavily promoted as "fat burners," although as unregulated substances they could vanish tomorrow. Many online weight-loss supplement sites offer their consumers reassurance that their products are safe because they're completely "natural" and not medications. Like ma huang, for instance, or arsenic. But even if using "natural" substances is safe, without rigorous scientific testing, contraindications for their use are unknown. And because these products aren't drugs, they likely have never been tested on human subjects.

WHAT'S IN A NAME

The difference between a drug and a supplement, according to the FDA, is this: A drug is prescribed to treat, prevent, or cure a specific condition or disease, while a dietary supplement *may* "help maintain" or "improve" a specific condition or disease. It is therefore far simpler to mix a few extracts together and market them over-the-counter as something that "*may* be the world's best weight-loss method" than to test a formula for years in the hope of providing evidence-based proof and winning FDA approval as a prescription drug that *will* cure obesity, that elusive holy grail of pharmaceutical companies.

Perhaps in reality there isn't an endless supply of herbal extracts that speed up the heart rate and metabolism, but it seems that way. Supplement manufacturers appear to be consistently able to come up with a new ingredient to replace whatever has been pulled from the shelves. It may be something old, like bladder wrack, or something new, like *Hoodia gordonii*, but scores of potential fat burners, appetite suppressants, and mood shifters are being tested to be ready for offering as substitutes for whatever is recalled next. Why all the recalls? The issue is that, although innocent until proven guilty may be exactly right in the halls of justice, it isn't when it comes to medicine, and a weight-loss "supplement" by any other name is just a drug that hasn't been put through the trials necessary to prove efficacy and safety.

Various weight-loss supplements have been associated with death for decades, and yet the Centers for Disease Control and Prevention reported that in 2006, Americans spent $1.3 billion on them. More than 20 percent of women and 10 percent of men had used them.

20

ANY OTHER OPTIONS, DOCTOR?

AMERICANS SPEND BILLIONS OF DOLLARS A YEAR ON DIET AND FITNESS PRODUCTS: Consider the popularity of television weight-loss competitions like *The Biggest Loser;* the wide availability of health club classes of every variety; the seemingly endless stream of diet books and articles; the meal services that deliver calorie-controlled portions right to your door; and the plethora of over-the-counter pills, prescription drugs, online support groups, and low-fat, low-carb, fat-free, and sugar-free foods. And yet in spite of all of this—and perhaps because of it—two-thirds of America is overweight.

One hundred years ago a few extra pounds were considered money in the bank, offering a little extra protection against infectious diseases. And they may well be thought of that way again. But if the pounds keep compounding and overweight progresses unchecked to obesity and then morbid obesity, there are only two options other than lifestyle change—bariatric surgery and prescription drugs. The first option is almost always guaranteed to work.

MAKING YOUR STOMACH SMALLER

The most drastic weight-loss solution—bariatric surgery—is recommended only for obese men and women with body mass indexes (BMIs) of greater than 35 who have weight-related illnesses such as diabetes and for those with BMIs of more than 40 without weight-related health

179

conditions. (About 5 percent of Americans have BMIs of greater than 40.) Though the procedure is often said to be dangerous, an analysis of almost 14,000 postoperative patients concluded that mortality is rare; another large study placed it at 0.25 percent. And the surgery is overwhelmingly effective. The World Health Organization (WHO) stated in a 2008 bulletin that there is "strong evidence that non-surgical treatment among subjects with severe or morbid obesity is insufficient," adding that bariatric surgery gives "good long term results . . . and improvement of quality of life." The largest study to date is the Swedish Obese Subjects Study, which followed 4,047 people for 2 years and 1,703 people for 10 years, with the groups split between those who achieved weight loss through surgery and those who used a combination of diet and exercise. The study found that bariatric surgery is the most viable method currently available for the very obese. Additionally, for patients with type 2 diabetes, the "recovery" rate for those who underwent surgery was significantly better in both the 2- and the 10-year groups.

More than 200,000 bariatric operations were performed in the United States in 2007—10 times more than took place in 1997.

The procedure most often performed is laparoscopic Roux-en-Y gastric bypass. A surgeon sections off a small pouch of the patient's stomach and connects it directly to the jejunum of his or her small intestine, thus bypassing the remainder of the stomach and the duodenum, the first part of the small intestine. Calorie absorption is limited because the pouch can hold very little food. Some patients also are unable to tolerate sugar. In 2008, CBS's *60 Minutes* aired a piece on the procedure that featured a panel of eight formerly diabetic and obese men and women. After undergoing the surgery, all became significantly thinner, exhibited no symptoms of diabetes, no longer craved sweets, and were extremely satisfied with the results. A surgeon (interviewed by Lesley Stahl) said that he expected his patients to end up about one-third lighter than their presurgery weight, but added that a severely obese person will probably never be thin (which suggests there may be a metabolic component to extreme obesity). He claimed the procedure has an 85 to 90 percent success rate and a mortality rate of 1 in 1,000 operations.

Laparoscopic adjustable gastric banding (inserting what's called a Lap-Band) is a simpler and less expensive option that doesn't involve and is somewhat less effective than surgery.

These procedures are expensive (gastric bypass surgery costs at least $25,000), but insurance companies often cover the cost, reasoning that the weight loss will lessen the high cost of future medical treatments.

Technological advances such as laparoscopy have made bariatric surgery much safer than it initially was, although negative results have been reported. Some patients suffer from physical side effects like nausea after eating, and others grapple with psychological struggles including depression and addictive behavior such as drinking or gambling that may replace overeating. Vitamin deficiencies are also common and are treated with supplements. It is a drastic lifestyle change for those who once lived to eat but now are forced to eat less to live.

The success rate for these surgeries is less than 100 percent because some people drink highly caloric beverages instead of eating the large quantities of food their stomachs can no longer hold, whereas others eat enough to stretch the remaining functional portion of their stomachs over time until they are once again able to tolerate excessive caloric intake. Some patients even manage to regain most or all of the weight they lost.

But complications and weight gain are rare, and the benefits are great. For example, WHO reports an 89 percent reduction in the risk of premature death and an 82 percent reduction in cardiovascular-related illness. However, this is an option only for the severely obese. To these patients, a physician is able to offer a "cure," but what about someone who just needs to lose 20 pounds?

IS THERE A PRESCRIPTION FOR WILLPOWER?

There was a time when certain doctors would prescribe antibiotics for the common cold, even though they knew the pills would do nothing to fight a virus. Eventually, it was discovered that the overuse of antibiotics in the general population was helping to create strains of antibiotic-resistant bacteria. But until that time, the drugs satisfied the patient's (and perhaps the doctor's) need to *do something*.

Many physicians are more comfortable with suggesting to patients that they take medicine than they are with discussing nutrition, and "eat less and exercise more" doesn't seem like much of a solution, especially if the doctor himself could stand to lose a few pounds. According to the Centers for Disease Control and Prevention, 58 percent of obese patients are never offered any advice about weight loss.

Whether or not obesity is a disease in and of itself or a chronic condition that may lead to a wide range of other diseases has been debated for decades. It is an interesting argument, because there are healthy obese people and unhealthy thin people, and obesity may contribute to disease in some, but not others. Extensive research that has been conducted to determine if certain individuals are genetically predisposed to being overweight or obese has examined metabolic, hormonal, and neurological factors. The most current evidence suggests that "for most people," obesity is "probably not" the result of a metabolic defect, but rather of "behavioral and environmental factors such as an unhealthy diet and decreased physical activity." In other words, after more than 100 years of research, the consensus is that most but not all people are obese because they eat too much and move too little.

It is thus possible that for a minority of overweight individuals, a hormonal issue such as hypothyroidism, enlarged fat cells, or another yet unknown factor has predisposed them to gaining and maintaining excess weight from the time they were in the womb. Recent research has centered on the classification of fat cells into categories of white and brown. Brown fat cells, which darken as they turn triglycerides into heat by oxidation, were until very recently thought to exist as a way to keep babies cozy and warm and then disappear after infancy. Adult humans either had no brown fat cells or the cells were irrelevant.

However, new imaging techniques recently led to the discoveries that adults do have brown fat cells and that thin people have more than those who are overweight, and that overweight people have more than the obese. Since the function of the brown cells is to regulate body temperature by burning glucose, it is theorized that brown fat cells introduced into an overweight adult might cause the white fat cells to dissolve. Research on whether this fat burner living inside us all may be useful as an obesity

182

remedy is proceeding cautiously, however, because the greatest numbers of brown fat cells are found in people with hyperthyroidism and cancer. Still, it is an intriguing concept.

However, if obesity is categorized as a disease, developing an effective remedy seems obligatory from a public health standpoint. It must have been a great relief for doctors when they were finally able to offer their patients prescriptions.

THE GREEKS CALL IT *LEPTOS*

In 1994, there was considerable excitement in the world of obesity research. Mice that had been genetically engineered to be obese* became slim when injected with leptin, an appetite- and metabolism-regulating hormone discovered at Rockefeller University in New York City by Jeffrey Friedman, MD, PhD, and his colleagues. It seemed plausible that if humans were injected with leptin (from the Greek word *leptos,* or "thin"), they might have the same results as the mice, and the biotechnology firm Amgen bought the patent.

But research was unable to prove that obese humans need more leptin. Instead, it appeared that heavy people produce so much of it that their brains become resistant to the hormone's signals. Although leptin research has so far proven unsuccessful in terms of finding an obesity cure, it has led to numerous other experiments into what are called the adipocyte-secreted hormones. These adipose (fat) cells, once believed to be no more than storage bins for fat, are now known to produce a wide variety of hormones that regulate appetite. This is one big Pandora's box of possibilities, and extensive research has been devoted to discovering whether a particular molecule might be a predictor of future obesity, or perhaps even the key to a way to lose weight effortlessly. This has been unsuccessful to date, likely because no single hormone is responsible, and the combinations that could be responsible are vast.

---

* Yes, this is possible. Many different types of "knockout mice" have been bred. They are called that not because of their inevitable fate, but because they have been genetically modified—that is, a gene has been knocked out or altered. Mice have also been genetically modified to be slim, but 70 percent of them die prematurely.

HOW MUCH ARE A FEW LESS POUNDS WORTH?

There are currently only two weight-loss drugs on the market that have FDA approval, and they are barely effective. Orlistat works by preventing the body from absorbing as much as one-third of consumed fat, albeit with a lot of what you may recall were olestra's unpleasant side effects—flatulence, diarrhea, stomach pains, and occasional "staining" of underwear. Considering this high cost of personal discomfort, it is relatively ineffectual, with weight loss averaging only a few pounds more than would be eliminated by a yearlong diet and exercise regimen. Orlistat is available by prescription as Xenical and sold over the counter as Alli (pronounced AL-eye, as in a supportive friend). Alli is a reduced-strength version of Xenical, and so the additional weight lost after a year of Alli as opposed to a year of diet and exercise alone is only about 5 pounds or less.

The FDA has been tracking safety issues related to these products. Between 1999 and 2008, there were 32 reports of serious injury to the liver and six of liver failure.

DIET-PILL REDUX

The other FDA-approved weight-loss drug is sibutramine, available by prescription under the trade name Meridia. It suppresses appetite by inhibiting the uptake of the brain hormones serotonin and norepinephrine (also called noradrenaline), so it is what is called a serotonin-norepinephrine reuptake inhibitor, or SNRI. Serotonin creates a sense of calm, whereas norepinephrine generates a feeling of excitement or stimulation. Chemically, sibutramine is related to Redux and fen-phen. There is a lot of controversy surrounding the drug, and it was recently taken off the market in Italy. Its side effects include high blood pressure and an increased heart rate. It is not very effective, either, with only a modest weight loss in excess of what one would accomplish with diet and exercise alone.

The conclusion about the currently available drugs is that their minimal benefits do not outweigh their risks. These high risks and low rewards render them neither worthless nor very valuable to the public or to the pharmaceutical companies desperately seeking to crack the obesity code.

Sanofi-Aventis expected to have great success with the drug rimonabant (available in Europe as Acomplia) and hyped it as a multipurpose miracle pill that would control overeating and alcohol abuse and help people stop smoking. The FDA denied it US approval in 2007 after five people in a trial of 36,000 committed suicide. It was pulled from the European market the following year. The pharmaceutical companies Merck and Pfizer immediately discontinued trials on their versions of the drug, which is now suspected of causing anxiety and depression. This should have been no surprise: The pill was to have been the first in a new class of diet drugs that worked by inhibiting the receptors that produce feelings of delight. Why eat chocolate cake if you don't enjoy it? The problem, for now, is that there is no way to segregate the pleasure receptors for food (or anything else) from those for other pleasurable experiences. So something that suppresses the happiness that comes with a hot fudge sundae will also suck the joy out of life.

WHAT'S LEFT?

As the obesity rate increases in the United States and many other developed countries, the prize for stopping it also grows. The person who is able to grasp the elusive golden key will have decoded the combination of elements that is needed to override what humans seem hardwired to do—overeat in a world where cheap, tasty food is ubiquitous.

Although sibutramine is relatively ineffective, scientists at the Danish company NeuroSearch are studying adding another neurotransmitter, dopamine, to the serotonin and norepinephrine formula, and so far the results have been promising. A small trial showed an average weight loss of approximately 10 percent in obese patients receiving 0.5 or 1 milligram over 24 weeks—more than twice the weight loss seen with sibutramine. Blood pressure was not elevated, nor was there an increased risk of depression. Reported side effects included only the minor concerns of nausea, dry mouth, and insomnia, and a larger trial is under way.

NAVIGATING THE CHEMISTRY OF THE BRAIN

Eating an orange is preferable to taking a vitamin C pill, because the fruit has fiber and more nutrients than we are perhaps even aware of and it's likely that they all work together synergistically to nourish us. There is still a great deal to be discovered about nutrition. Brain chemistry is an even newer science. Serotonin, dopamine, and norepinephrine were not identified until less than 75 years ago, and there are undoubtedly neurotransmitters still to be discovered. Some may even be integral parts of the weight-loss solution.

Finding a pill that will control appetite is an elusive thing. Hormones work together to form memories, create feelings of satisfaction, and allow the emotional pain that comes with trauma to diminish, and this may help to explain why food is so much more than just a fuel supply, and why those few who, like Nathan Pritikin, enjoy more spartan diets are the few who never have to diet. For the rest of us, there may well be a billion-dollar formula someday that won't tinker with the most basic needs and emotions of the human mind but can still suppress the desire to eat the foods we love. But while the pharmaceutical companies race toward a safe and effective means of appetite control, food industry scientists are researching something completely different. Their goal—to find ways to make us eat as much as possible—is much easier to achieve.

21

ARE WE JUST *REALLY* HUNGRY?

AS WE ENTER THE 2ND DECADE OF THE NEW MILLENNIUM, THERE'S NO QUESTION THAT Americans are heavier than ever. We also seem to be more depressed than ever—the use of antidepressants doubled between 1996 and 2005. (Comedian Jimmy Fallon aptly quipped on his late-night comedy-talk show in August 2009 that the only people who aren't depressed are the ones manufacturing the drugs.) It is ironic that some antidepressants—and other widely prescribed medications, as we'll explore later—can increase users' weights, while some weight-loss medications have been taken off the market because they result in anxiety and depression.

Some recent studies have also suggested that the food we are eating is making us fat *and* depressed. Foods rich in omega-3 fatty acids, which are lacking in the typical American diet, may act as antidepressants. (Good sources include wild salmon, herring, sardines, meat and dairy products from grass-fed animals, walnuts, flaxseed oil, wild greens, and eggs from free-range chickens.) These omega-3 fatty acids that are so essential to our health and well-being are not found in processed foods, fast foods, and products derived from factory-farmed animals; in other words, most of us aren't getting nearly enough of them. According to Susan Allport, author of *The Queen of Fats*, omega-3s are the most abundant fats in the world. They are found in the green leaves of plants, which are consumed in abundance by wild fish and grazing animals. It is these nutrient-dense leaves that kept Vilhjalmur Stefansson in such good health on his all-meat Inuit diet.

Ideally, plant-based omega-3s should be in balance with omega-6 fatty acids, which are derived from seeds. Everything was in harmony, according to Allport, until corn and soy began to be planted "fencerow to fencerow." At that point, the huge surpluses resulted in corn and soy oils becoming ubiquitous in our diet. They were believed to be healthy (unsaturated!), they were cheap, and they became ingredients in snack foods, cookies, crackers, and fast foods. At the same time, omega-3 fatty acids became scarce because animals were no longer allowed to graze and seafood began being farmed. Cattle, chickens, and fish were all fed corn and soy, and we ended up with a diet very rich in omega-6 fatty acids and deficient in omega-3s. That imbalance is suspected of being at the foundation of multiple health issues, including hormonal and neurological problems and obesity.

BIG WEIGHT LOSS

In turn, weight management is a $55 billion industry in the United States. In January 2010, Standard and Poor's (S&P) recommended buying shares of Weight Watchers International because of the "rising trend of obesity." But the investment analysts at S&P assessed the risk profile for this investment as "medium" rather than "low" because "so many approaches to weight loss have been created and marketed." We are, as a nation, feeding for-profit industries when we overeat. There's Big Food and Big Weight Loss, with Big Pharma straining to get an ever-larger piece of the pie, and not just by trying to find that still-elusive weight-loss drug, but also from all the medications they sell to cure or control obesity-related diseases and conditions, such as type 2 diabetes and high blood pressure.

Since 2004 the nonprofit and nonpartisan Robert Wood Johnson Foundation has been publishing an annual report that analyzes obesity trends in the United States. The obesity rate did not decline in any state in 2008, but it increased in 23 of them. In 1980, 15 percent of US adults were obese; today, it is more than 33 percent.* Food is inexpensive and

---

* Adults with a body mass index (BMI) of 30 or higher are considered obese. BMI = weight in pounds divided by [height in inches squared] times 703. Calculators are easy to find and use online: http://www.nhlbisupport.com/bmi.

plentiful. And even though most of us know better, we're still eating too much of it.

Excess weight often accumulates gradually—no one becomes obese overnight. A few extra calories each day add up to a few extra pounds each year. (Curiously, this fact is still debated after 100 years of evidence.) The question is: Why are so many people—many of whom are well aware of the consequences of their food choices—eating more than they need to? And why can't they stop?

BIG FAT PROFITS

David Kessler, physician, attorney, and head of the FDA during both the Bill Clinton and George H. W. Bush administrations, offers an intriguing explanation in his best-selling 2009 book, *The End of Overeating*. Kessler believes that the food industry has successfully created a nation of addicts unable to resist the high-sugar, high-fat, high-salt combinations that food technologists have developed to entice us. We are Snow Whites tempted by poison Applebee's, chomping our way through the Cheesecake Factory and row after row of processed snacks.

The world's great chefs know how to turn "craveability" into an art form. At L'Arpège, long considered one of the finest restaurants in Paris, Chef Alain Passard begins every diner's meal with an unforgettable gift: a petite poached egg yolk served in its shell, topped with a tiny amount of crème fraiche, sherry vinegar, maple syrup, and fleur de sel. Luckily, expense and availability prevent these memorably irresistible little snacks from becoming addictive; otherwise, they would be consumed daily by the dozens. This is the blissful plate state known as craveability that food technicians aim for, except their versions are highly processed and cheap, and barely resemble actual food.

Kessler says that our neurons—our brain cells—are encoded to react to certain food characteristics. A neuron may respond to texture, temperature, smell, or, most important of all, taste. When they are stimulated by foods created to be "highly palatable," brain cells release endorphins into our bloodstreams. This is similar to the response created by morphine, heroin, exercise, or orgasm. Over time, many people become unable to resist the foods that lead to this state of euphoria and desire them more than they are able to control themselves. Irresistible items differ from one person's plate (or bucket) to the next, but Big Food has plenty of tricks up its sleeve to keep customers eating plenty and coming back for seconds.

Food industry technologists have moved quickly to capitalize on new breakthroughs in brain research, developing innovative ways to get us to eat more of their products. Their success in this is as deviously impressive as it is arguably immoral. It also underscores just how much easier it is to gain weight in a land of processed plenty than it is to lose it.

As President Calvin Coolidge said shortly before the Great Depression, "The business of America is business." The business of producing and processing most of our foods and, yes, of packaging, marketing, and selling it to consumers exemplifies the tenets of old-fashioned American capitalism. They wouldn't keep selling if we didn't keep buying.

But if we know these things—that the food we are eating is nutritionally bankrupt, that the food manufacturers manipulate us into eating more—why do we continue to eat the way we do? "Tell me what you eat, and I will tell you what you are," challenged French lawyer and *Physiology of Taste* author Anthelme Brillat-Savarin in 1825. What are we, then, if we are eating Hardee's Monster Thickburgers—1,420-calorie concoctions of bacon, cheese, and mayonnaise on top of a burger inside a buttered bun? Are we depressed because we weigh too much in a country where thinness reigns supreme despite the fact that the majority of Americans are overweight? Are we eating to comfort ourselves over the things we cannot control—the economy, job security, war, politics?

Or have we simply been transformed into robotic feeding machines programmed to seek out and consume as much cheap, delicious, salty, fatty, sugary food as we can get our hands on?

22

WHAT EPIDEMIC?

WHAT IF, AS NEUROSCIENTIST PAUL ERNSBERGER, PHD; ATTORNEY PAUL CAMPOS; and physiologist Glenn Gaesser, PhD, suggest, "the so-called 'obesity epidemic' is largely an illusion"? There is no epidemic, they claim, because the scientific data doesn't support its existence. Nor, they contend, do the data provide evidence-based proof that "overweight and obesity are major contributors to mortality" or disease, or that long-term weight loss is beneficial. The epidemic may be a scam manufactured by the same people who manufacture diet food, diet pills, and diet products. The high mortality rate associated with obesity, these contrarians suggest, may in fact be inflated due to the increased use of deadly over-the-counter diet pills.

The problem with this line of reasoning—that we should stop the war on fat not because we surrender, but because there is no enemy—is that there is, in fact, a tremendous body of research linking obesity to life-threatening diseases and shortened life spans. The consequences of obesity simply can't be argued away, no matter how appealing it may be to imagine it is all just a conspiracy to sell more diet pills and running shoes.

However, it is valid to question the meaning of "overweight." Any culture's definition of "optimal" is ultimately determined by society, and this year's "pleasingly plump" or "stylishly stout" can become next year's "fat." As evident in the seemingly arbitrary shifts in the Metropolitan Life Insurance Company's weight charts in 1942, 1959, and 1983, flimsy evidence can sometimes be used to determine an ideal. Definitions of "overweight" or "underweight" are mercurial—so it seems rational to conclude that having a BMI of 26 or 27 (instead of the coveted 24) should be no cause for alarm. For example, a recent study finds that the life expectancy of subjects who

191

are categorized as overweight but are physically active enough to maintain large amounts of lean muscle is roughly equal to that of those who are thin but not physically fit. Some research has even suggested that people who are overweight (but not obese) are likely to live *longer* than those of normal weight if they are physically active. The "fit and fat" argument was made by contrarian Gaesser using evidence the Cooper Institute for Aerobics Research in Dallas collected on 9,777 men over a 5-year period. Once again, men who were the least fit (not the heaviest) had the highest age-adjusted death rate, and those who were the most fit (not the thinnest) had the lowest. In yet another study, the physical data of 11,326 adults were analyzed over a 12-year period; in the end, scientists found that slightly overweight nonsmokers were 17 percent *less* likely to die than normal-weight nonsmokers. The researchers theorized that a bit of extra weight might actually be protective against infectious diseases, especially in the elderly—as long as they also make use of the many medications and procedures that are readily available to fight obesity-related health problems.

So, one may conclude, as long as they take the right drugs and are willing to undergo any necessary surgeries, the one-third of Americans who are labeled overweight (as opposed to the one-third who are labeled obese) may not have to worry about the impact of their weight on their overall quality (and duration) of life. If they're physically active, they might not be at increased risk for heart disease, diabetes, stroke, cancer, or Alzheimer's disease. In other words, it is reasonable to assume that someone carrying a few extra pounds who eats a mostly healthy diet and who exercises on a regular basis will not suffer because he or she does not have the "correct" BMI for his or her height. BMI and other measurements are most effectively used to evaluate populations, not individuals, and they serve as very rough guidelines.

BUT MOST PEOPLE AREN'T FIT

The problem with the "fit and fat" argument is that often, overweight people (and normal-weight and underweight people) aren't in the best physical shape. But it's the combination of the two—overweight *and* unfit—that puts them at a higher risk for complications from disease. In addition, excess weight usually results from eating too many processed foods with high "craveability,"* rather than lots of nutrient-dense fruits, vegetables, and whole grains that protect against disease. And overweight, if left unchecked, often leads to obesity and ill health.

DO THESE PILLS MAKE ME LOOK FAT?

While considerable advances have been made in medicines to treat diabetes, high cholesterol, high blood pressure, and depression, a side effect of many of them is weight gain. Two drugs for type 2 diabetes, pioglitazone (Actos) and rosiglitazone (Avandia and Avandamet), result in gains of up to 17 pounds during an intensive 3-month treatment, and users of the diabetes medications glimepiride (Amaryl), glipizide (Glucotrol), glipizide with metformin (Metaglip), and glyburide with metformin (Glucovance) can gain up to 11 pounds in 3 to 12 months' time. Drugs for bipolar disorder have been reported to cause "drastic weight gain and metabolic changes," especially in children. There is also evidence that the selective serotonin reuptake inhibitors prescribed for depression result in an average 15 to 20 pounds of weight gain. Depression and obesity may intersect in other ways. Since the 1960s, it has been theorized that some depressed people self-medicate with carbohydrates, because that nutrient elevates levels of serotonin in the brain. Ironically, being overweight in a never-too-thin society can be depressing enough to make you want another piece of cake, which is full of fast-release carbohydrates that lead to deeper depression, which results in your physician prescribing medication that results in weight gain. This is in no way to suggest that these medications aren't necessary for many people. However, it might explain why Redux wasn't all that effective, and why Meridia isn't either.

ONE MORE TIME: IS OBESITY REALLY HAZARDOUS TO YOUR HEALTH?

Although the argument can be (and has been) made that you can be a bit overweight and still be healthy, it is doubtful that anyone would argue that

---

* The French have a word for this: *malbouffe*, defined as a poor diet that has a negative impact on one's health.

overweight, left unchecked, is a good thing. There is no Faustian bargain that allows you to remain very obese, happy, vigorous, and healthy in exchange for just a few years less of life. The data may indicate, for example, that 60 extra pounds correlates with a 5- to 12-year reduction in life span, but it isn't quite that simple. Obesity results in having a much higher risk of developing a wide variety of diseases, only some of which are controllable by medication, and all of which have very negative impacts on quality of life. There is no certainty that the loss will be just a few years of life or that one's final years will be productive and enjoyable, because the consequences of obesity-related diseases are severe. Certainly, the future is unknown, and any given person—fat or thin—could die tomorrow. But the odds of living fully and actively for as long as possible are greatly diminished by obesity.

FIT, FAT, AND HEALTHY

There is evidence, as mentioned, that being fit has a greater impact on health than being thin does, and compelling arguments support the notion that you can have a healthy lifestyle despite not conforming to the compartmentalized charts, scales, and tape measures used to define "health." One new way of looking in the mirror is via the prism of Health at Every Size. Linda Bacon, PhD, a physiologist, nutritionist, and proponent of this philosophy, recommends that we ignore the cultural attributes ascribed to weight and size and respect our bodies enough to stop trying to force them to become shapes they were never meant to be. The idea is to concentrate on optimal health, not clothing size. It is a terrific notion for people who beat themselves up for being a bit overweight, but certainly not for the 33 percent of obese Americans. Here, the risks seem irrefutable. An obese person will likely have a tragically diminished life span, as well as a seriously compromised quality of life.

While the roles of food and pharmaceutical manufacturers may be under debate, the statistics don't lie: We are a nation with an epidemic proportion of obese individuals, many of whom suffer from serious diseases as a result of their unhealthy weights. Obesity cannot be wished away as fantasy.

PART FIVE

WEIGHING IN ON

THE FUTURE

23

THE MYSTERIOUS
CASE OF THE DIET
DOCTOR

ON APRIL 7, 2003, THERE WAS A SNOWSTORM IN NEW YORK CITY, WHICH, COMBINED with the unseasonably cold weather, made getting around the city streets difficult and dangerous. Two days earlier, Robert C. Atkins, the most famous diet doctor of the 20th century, had decided to sell his 80 percent share of Atkins Nutritionals for $533 million. He was thinking of retiring to Palm Beach, Florida, where he and his wife were renovating a large home. The business seemed to be worth at least that much, if not more. So many people were "on Atkins" that his processed food line was not only available in most supermarkets, it was also given prominent display space. The brand seemed to be ubiquitous.

Early in the morning of April 8, the 72-year-old doctor set out on foot from his apartment in Midtown Manhattan to go to the nearby Atkins Center for Complementary Medicine at 152 East 55th Street. As he approached the entrance, he fell to the ground. Unconscious and bleeding heavily from wounds on the back of his head, he was recognized by an employee, Keith Berkowitz, MD, who called an ambulance and accompanied him to the closest hospital, Weill Cornell Medical Center. Atkins slipped into a coma en route and never regained consciousness. Nine days later, his wife Veronica agreed to remove him from life support. No autopsy was performed, and the body was cremated.

197

There was tremendous controversy surrounding his death. Before he committed suicide, Nathan Pritikin had given clear instructions that he wanted an autopsy to be performed on his body—and it had provided evidence that his diet was effective. Veronica Atkins, on the other hand, refused to release any of her husband's medical records. Robert Atkins may have collapsed due to a heart attack or a stroke—but she firmly stated that her husband's death had been nothing more than an accident. He had simply slipped on a patch of ice.

Months later, Neal Barnard, MD, professor at George Washington University's medical school, head of the Physicians Committee for Responsible Medicine, and an Atkins critic, requested a copy of the death certificate. Though he wasn't Atkins's attending physician and never should have received the confidential medical records, he did, and he forwarded the certificate to the *Wall Street Journal*. According to the published medical examiner's report, Atkins had suffered from a heart attack, congestive heart failure, and hypertension. In addition, he weighed 258 pounds at the time of his death, which, on his 6-foot frame, was a great deal of weight. If his high-fat diet had failed him—and there was now a lot of reason to believe that it had—his empire, certainly, seemed in danger of collapse.

This big story was made bigger when New York City's mayor, Michael Bloomberg, made some unfortunate remarks about Atkins's death at a luncheon for firefighters. Believing that his microphone was off, Bloomberg used profanity to convey his opinion of the "slip and fall" excuse, saying the real reason the doctor had died was because he was fat. He went on to describe a fund-raiser he had attended at the home of Robert and Veronica in Southampton. The food was so bad, he said, "I took one appetizer and I had to spit it into my napkin." His comments made it onto the evening news.

Veronica Atkins appeared on television to refute Bloomberg's theory about her husband's death, defend her caterer, and demand an apology. Bloomberg eventually did say he was sorry, and he invited her out for a steak dinner, no potatoes. She never went.

The widow and Atkins's associates continued to deny there was any health-related reason for his death. It was known that he had been hospitalized for cardiac arrest in 2002 after being revived with CPR, but Atkins had made a public statement contending that he had an enlarged heart, which Veronica said she thought had resulted from a sinus infection. His cardiologist and employee, Patrick Fratellone, MD, told *New York* magazine that his late boss's coronary arteries were "30 to 40 percent blocked" and added that he thought that was "pretty good for a man who eats that much fat." Finally, Veronica Atkins conceded that her husband did, in fact, have some coronary artery disease during the last 3 years of his life, including some new blockage, had been on heart-rhythm medication, and had taken about 50 dietary supplements a day.

Atkins representatives continued to deny heart disease had been implicated in his cause of death, maintaining that Atkins had weighed only 195 pounds when he was admitted to the hospital and that the intravenous fluids that he had received had caused his body to swell. The $1.25 billion low-carb food industry, which had been projected to double in 2004, was instead beginning to dwindle. The company's sales fell 32 percent between October and December in 2004. Sales continued to free-fall, plummeting 50 percent in the first half of 2005. Atkins Nutritionals filed for bankruptcy protection later that year. Veronica Atkins had closed the clinic in October 2003 and moved to Palm Beach, Florida.

When he published his first diet book in 1972, Robert Atkins had sententiously written, "Martin Luther King had a dream. I, too, have one. I dream of a world where no one has to diet." More than 30 years later, his dream was still unfulfilled. Millions of people had tried his plan, and more people than ever needed to lose weight.

COPY CARBS

It had been a good business decision to sell Atkins Nutritionals in 2003. After all, Vilhjalmur Stefansson's nearly identical approach to weight loss was called a "scientific milestone" in the 1950s. "High fat was riding high," Stefansson wrote, "and so was I with it, proudly. But pride goeth before a fall, and what a fall was there, my countrymen!"

Robert Atkins had been riding a similar high after a 2002 *New York Times Magazine* cover article by science writer Gary Taubes argued that maybe fat didn't make you fat after all and that staying away from carbohydrates might be a credible solution. The American Heart Association (AHA) even invited Atkins to be a guest speaker.

Though his processed foods business was soaring, Atkins knew that being a superstar in the diet business was fleeting at best. He had watched his sales plummet during the low-fat craze of the '80s and dealt with competition from another contender for the low-carb-diet crown, cardiologist Arthur Agatston, MD, who had already sold 5 million copies of his *South Beach Diet.*

South Beach was a low-*bad*-carb, high-*good*-fat diet that emphasized high-fiber complex carbohydrates like vegetables and whole grains and fats from olive oil and fish. Saturated fats, white rice, white bread, white potatoes, and pastas were discouraged, along with desserts and sugary soft drinks. In other words, it was a diet the American Medical Association and the AHA could endorse. With lots of simple and heart-healthy recipes from Floridian chefs, it was replacing Atkins as the Big Diet for the new millennium.

Early in 2004, the director of research for Atkins tried to regain some market share from South Beach by placing a new emphasis on lowering the number of calories allowed from saturated fats in the diet. The Atkins dietitians had been traveling the country preaching this reduction for the previous 5 years, but only to health care professionals. They had neglected to put it in the *"Completely Updated!"* 2002 edition of the book, because, as they put it, they didn't want to confuse the public. Suddenly, people on Atkins *couldn't* eat all the butter, bacon, pork rinds, and steaks they wanted. Game, set, match.

Atkins's top employees were in a race to assume their boss's place in the diet world after his death, and they all tried to distance themselves from the high-fat Atkins image. "I'm moving to where Atkins would have gone," announced Fred Pescatore, MD, the Atkins associate medical director who had opened his own clinic and was about to publish *The Hamptons Diet.* Based on the Mediterranean Diet devised by Ancel Keys, Pescatore's plan featured unsaturated fats, whole grains, lots of fruits and vegetables, and organic foods and emphasized a "secret ingredient"—macadamia nut oil that you could buy directly from him. The book's Web site stresses that his plan is *the* way for the "rich, indulgent, and thin" Hamptons crowd to maintain their litheness.

Internist Keith Berkowitz had been Atkins's business director for only 2 months on the day he discovered him bleeding on the sidewalk, but he claimed that he had been hired to take over the business. To that end, he quickly opened his own diet center, took 200 patients with him, and cofounded a low-carb food company. Patrick Fratellone, Atkins's cardiologist and chief medical director—and the man who blew the whistle on Atkins's clogged arteries—opened yet another facility focusing on integrative medicine. The Upper East Side of Manhattan may have lost Robert C. Atkins, but it retained most of his acolytes, who were quick to throw the more controversial parts of the Atkins diet under the wheels of the ice cream truck.

24

GENETICS, CHEMISTRY, AND A PLASTIC WORLD

IN 1960, 13 PERCENT OF ALL AMERICANS WERE OBESE. BY 1980, THAT NUMBER HAD RISEN to 15 percent, and over the next 20 years, it doubled. Currently, it is at 34.3 percent and holding. That's good news, because although there is no evidence that the rate is decreasing, it does appear to have reached a plateau.

The bad news is that only 32 percent of the adult population—and only 28 percent of American men—are currently at what is considered to be a healthy weight. A "healthy weight," as defined by the World Health Organization (WHO), is a BMI of less than 25, because 25 is the cutoff point beyond which mortality increases, although, as previously mentioned, there is evidence that a physically active person with a BMI of between 25 and 29 might be at a weight that is "healthy" for him or her. Ironically, when WHO first implemented the BMI scale in the 1980s, it was used as an indicator for at-risk *under*weight populations in developing nations, not for what WHO now refers to as "globesity."

More than 400 million people in the world are obese, which is defined as having a BMI of 30 or higher.* Though it's true that we may be feeding the worldwide problem by exporting many of our dietary preferences around the globe, the most current OECD *Factbook* data indicate that much of the world still resists assimilating the American diet. Japan, France, and Italy, for example—countries with distinguished and revered culinary traditions—have low rates of obesity compared to much of the rest of the Western world.

In addition to having an increased risk of early death from coronary heart disease, stroke, diabetes (70 percent of people who have type 2 diabetes are overweight or obese), and sleep apnea, there is a suspected correlation between obesity and cancers of the breast, uterus, cervix, colon, esophagus, pancreas, prostate, and kidney. Not to mention lower-back pain, gallbladder disease, osteoarthritis, and the psychological challenges of being overweight in a country that puts a very high premium on being slim.

It is beyond dispute that taking in more calories than you expend will result in weight gain, just as Wilbur Atwater insisted more than 100 years ago. It also seems evident that it doesn't make any difference if those extra calories come from carbohydrates, proteins, or fats. Eating fewer calories by cutting back on bread *or* butter makes no difference; you'll lose weight. If Robert Atkins and Nathan Pritikin were still alive, they could argue about whether low carb beats low fat for the next 100 years, but they would be wasting our time. The people of Japan and Korea, which have the lowest rates of obesity in the developed world, have a traditional diet that is one of the lowest in fat, but the cuisines of Italy, France, Germany, Switzerland, Austria, and Sweden are not particularly low fat, yet their citizens still have very low rates of obesity. Calories matter.

---

* Obesity rates, from highest to lowest, according to data from the Organisation for Economic Co-Operation and Development (OECD), as published in the *OECD Factbook 2009,* for populations ages 15 and above (2006 or latest available data) are as follows: United States (34 percent), Mexico (30 percent), New Zealand (26 percent), United Kingdom (24 percent), Greece (22 percent), Australia (22 percent), Canada (18 percent), Spain (15 percent), Finland (14 percent), Germany (14 percent), Ireland (13 percent), Austria (12 percent), Sweden (11 percent), France (10 percent), Italy (10 percent), Norway (8 percent), Switzerland (7 percent), Japan (4 percent), Korea (4 percent).

GENETICALLY PROGRAMMED

Portrait galleries are filled with the images of robust, well-heeled people of other eras. Peter Paul Rubens, so well known for his depictions of plump subjects that his name inspired the adjective "Rubenesque," painted in the 17th century. Shakespeare's Prince Hal insulted Sir John Falstaff by calling him a "huge hill of flesh" at about the same time. Hippocrates, born circa 460 BC, clinically observed, "Sudden death is more common in those who are naturally fat than in the lean." Stone Age drawings of the morbidly obese have been discovered.

That 13 percent of the US population who were obese in 1960 were neither part of an epidemic nor news; there have always been people who have a predilection for eating more than is strictly necessary if the calories are available. Not everyone trying to lose weight at the turn of the 20th century was doing it to be trendy. But there's a difference today. All of those cheap, delicious, readily available fattening foods, combined with our sedentary lifestyle, have made it easier to become overweight and obese. Certainly, there's too much on our collective plate. But there may be extenuating circumstances.

Some people have inherited an "obesity gene," that is, a gene that makes them particularly adept at storing fat. Preliminary research indicates that people with one variant of this gene weigh, on average, 6.6 pounds more than those who lack it. Those extra pounds were easier to keep off before our food supply became such a challenge to navigate and cheap and fattening foods became ubiquitous. There is evidence that almost 10 percent of morbidly obese individuals possess variants in the genes that control satiety, body weight, and metabolism—an indication that for many of them, genetics plays a more active role. If that's the case, it may explain why some people can't seem to lose weight no matter how little they eat, and even remain above their "healthy" weight after bariatric surgery. About 4 million Americans are currently categorized as morbidly obese, and genetic research may prove invaluable in determining why. For the rest of us, it seems safe to assume that it is a behavioral problem, not a change in our genetic makeup (which would typically take millennia to evolve) that has set in over the past 30 years. Our genes didn't make us fat—our lifestyles did.

THE BALANCE SCALE WEIGHS NATURE AND NURTURE

The Pima Indians, who live on both sides of the US–Mexican border, are often cited as an example of the impact of heredity versus the environment on body weight because the contrast between the two groups is so striking. Although their genetic makeup is essentially identical, the American Pimas, who live about halfway between Phoenix and Tucson, have far higher rates of obesity and type 2 diabetes than the Mexican Pima community. The US population's obesity rate of 69 percent is also higher than that found among the Mexican Pimas, the rest of the population of Arizona, and even the nation. The Mexican Pimas, who live in the Sierra Madre, are *not* overweight, and type 2 diabetes is rare.* Although both groups inherited the same "thrify" gene that causes their bodies to store fat in times of plenty as a hedge against famine, the diet and energy expenditure of the Mexican Pimas precludes morbid obesity, whereas those of the American Pimas encourages it. Interestingly, the American Pima Indians were not obese prior to World War II, when they still followed a lifestyle traditional to their culture.

DOES THIS SHOWER CURTAIN MAKE ME LOOK FAT?

In the 1967 film *The Graduate,* Dustin Hoffman plays Ben, a young man who has recently returned home to Los Angeles after graduating from college. He has absolutely no idea of what to do with the rest of his life. At the cocktail party where he meets Mrs. Elaine Robinson, a businessman and family friend gives him a piece of advice that became symbolic of a changing America: "I just want to say one word to you, just one word," the guy says earnestly. "Are you listening? *Plastics!* There's a great future in plastics."

---

* In comparison, 5.1 percent of the global population, 7.9 percent of the total US population, 7.1 percent of the Mexican Pimas, and 38 percent of the Arizona Pimas have type 2 diabetes. The average weight of a male Mexican Pima is 145 pounds; for a male American Pima, the average is 215 pounds.

Although plastics represented a horrifying future to Ben, the businessman was right. Plastics were becoming the stuff of food wraps, pacifiers, nonstick cookware, storage containers, baby bottles, and toys. Not a day goes by that we don't encounter plastic in one form or another.

Manhattan's Mount Sinai Medical Center recently published results of a study that linked obesity to phthalates—compounds found in plastics. Phthalates are absorbed by the body and may disrupt metabolism, and, it is theorized, cause early-onset puberty in girls. Urinalysis of 400 girls ages 9 to 11 revealed that the heaviest girls had the highest levels of phthalate metabolites in their systems and the thinnest had the least. A larger nationwide study of 100,000 children is under way to analyze the effects of plastics on metabolic function. In another recent study, Belgian scientists found that the children who were exposed in utero to the highest levels of PCBs—polychlorinated biphenyls—resulting from the chemical breakdown of pesticides became heavier infants. The Harvard School of Public Health has reported that obesity in infants ages 6 months and under has risen dramatically since 1980; researchers suspect a connection with phthalates or other chemical compounds that are transferred in utero or ingested, inhaled, or absorbed through the skin after birth. Phthalates are ubiquitous in lotions, toys, cosmetics, and plastic baby bottles. As if fat genes, sedentary lifestyles, and cheap, irresistible, high-calorie snacks created in labs by "food architects" weren't enough, the chemicals found in plastics and pesticides may predispose us to becoming fat even before we are born.

These chemicals, which are referred to as obesogens, are endocrine disruptors that trick the body into reacting as if the hormone estrogen has been released. This may flip a switch in a cell that makes it become an adipocyte—a fat cell—instead of another type of cell. Some drugs for diabetes also activate this receptor switch, called PPAR gamma, which is likely why many people gain weight while on diabetes medications.

Having superfluous fat cells may make your body use fewer calories as energy and store them as fat instead. This is all still theoretical, but it may help explain why an infant (for whom eating less and exercising more isn't really an option) living on breast milk might be obese and have great difficulty losing weight as he or she grows up.

According to the Children's Environmental Health Center at Mount Sinai Medical Center in New York City, more than 80,000 new chemicals have been developed since midcentury, and scientists are just beginning to discover the impacts these chemical cocktails have on our health.

25

THE 7 PERCENT SOLUTION

MANY AMERICAN PRESIDENTS AND THEIR FIRST LADIES HAVE DISPLAYED A PREFERENCE FOR wholesome foods. Laura Bush wanted organic, healthy meals for herself and her family; Hillary Clinton requested that high-quality products be used in the White House kitchen; and Dwight D. Eisenhower maintained a farm in Gettysburg, Pennsylvania, where he raised cattle and had a summer vegetable garden.

But none of them spoke of this often in public, perhaps to distance themselves from a perceived "elitist" association with healthy foods.

Issues of health care and the epidemic called obesity have brought food issues very much to the forefront of public awareness, and eating well may for the first time in a long time become a sign of good sense rather than a sign of a "health nut" or of weight-loss-fad lunacy.

The administration of President Barack Obama seems to be intent upon influencing and educating Americans about the virtues of healthy foods and healthy farms, from shopping at farmers' markets, to planting an organic garden on the White House grounds, to installing inexpensive hoop houses—rudimentary greenhouses—to ensure they have a supply of fresh, organic lettuces, carrots, and other crops throughout the winter. Michelle Obama's Healthy Kids Initiative is focusing on eliminating what she refers to as the major public health threat of childhood obesity. She believes that children and their parents will improve their diets if they are taught how to do so with compassion and humor, and if they are given realistic goals. Even if dissenters mock these obvious attempts to influence the way America eats, the Obamas are, at the very least, getting the nation talking about what's for dinner. Unless we begin to value our bodies and have both the information to make rational decisions and the skills to cook simple foods well, we will never reduce our collective weight. We need to coin an Americanized word for the French *malbouffe*. "Junk food" connotes KFC and Twinkies, but not all the rest of it—the sweetened cereals, sugary drinks, breakfast bars, salty snacks, and frozen desserts—the stuff that is the foundation of the obesity pyramid.

THE SIN TAX

Lulu Hunt Peters suggested levying an obesity tax in 1925. The idea of a "fat tax" on specific nutritionally empty products has emerged repeatedly in the last few years, only to be quashed every time by lobbyists from all of those giant industries that would be negatively affected.

There is no dispute that heavily taxing an unhealthy product has a powerful impact. *Smoking and Health: Report of the Advisory Committee to the Surgeon General of the Public Health Service* was published on Saturday, January 11, 1964. (A Saturday was chosen to minimize effects on the stock market and to maximize the opportunity for coverage in the Sunday newspapers.) That cigarette smoking is hazardous to your health wasn't really new information—in 1958, 44 percent of Americans said that they believed smoking caused cancer. But the groundbreaking report made it official, and by 1968, 78 percent of Americans believed that smoking was dangerous for their health. However, it was the higher taxes on every pack of cigarettes, along with new antismoking laws, that led to the dramatic decrease in smoking in America. In 1965, when the Centers for Disease Control and Prevention (CDC) began keeping records, 42.4 percent of the adult population smoked. As taxes increased, smoking continued to steadily decline. In 1987, the figure fell below 30 percent, and by 2007 less than 20 percent of adult Americans smoked. Cigarettes are currently taxed in all states on a discretionary basis (New York has the highest tax, at $2.75 per pack, while Virginia taxes its smokers a mere 30 cents per pack). The federal government now taxes every pack an additional $1.01, the result of the single largest federal tax hike on tobacco in US history—an increase of 62 cents per pack—that went into effect in April 2009. (The resulting revenues are being used to fund the State Children's Health Insurance Program, often called SCHIP.) Matthew McKenna, MD, director of the Office on Smoking and Health at the CDC, said he expects the federal tax hike to get at least 1 million more smokers to quit. The World Health Organization reports that for every 10 percent increase in the cigarette tax, there is a corresponding 4 percent decrease in consumption.

But tobacco is a single controlled substance, so can the same approaches to controlling its use be applied to foods? Food is food . . . or is it? Can a product that contains no nutritive benefit and provides no feeling of satiety really be categorized as a food? Is it logical that the price of a beverage that may contribute to health problems has increased by only 32 percent between 1983 and 2005, whereas other potentially harmful beverages, such as hard liquor, beer, and wine, are subject to "sin taxes"?

Each adult in America consumes, on average, about 1 million calories a year, and about 7 percent of those calories come from soft drinks made with caloric sweeteners. In 1980, before that cheap "floozy of the sugar world," as *Washington Post* nutrition columnist Sally Squires refers to high-fructose corn syrup, made upsizing extremely profitable and soda one of the least expensive things you could buy, about 3 percent of Americans' calories came from soft drinks. Decreasing our current rate of consumption by only 10 percent would save each of us an average of 7,000 calories (or 2 pounds) per person annually. Giving up sweetened beverages entirely could theoretically save an amazing 20 pounds in 1 year.

PUTTING FRUITS AND VEGETABLES BACK IN THE SHOPPING CART

In contrast to soda, the prices of fresh fruits have increased by 190 percent since 1980. The costs of fresh vegetables have increased by 144 percent.

If the price of a can of regular soda was doubled, consumption would undoubtedly decrease; it is not an addictive substance, and diet soda and other beverages are readily available alternatives. Since the empty calories derived from drinking sweetened sodas have been correlated with high triglycerides, low HDL (good) cholesterol, glucose intolerance, high blood pressure, and risk of coronary heart disease and diabetes, this would be a positive public health measure. As with the tobacco tax increase of 2009, the revenues could be directed toward funding health care and programs like the Healthy Kids Initiative. And the obesity rate—especially among children—would decline.

"COKE DIDN'T MAKE AMERICANS FAT"

"Americans need more exercise, not another tax," according to Muhtar Kent, the CEO of the Coca-Cola Company. Kent acknowledges that there is an obesity problem in our country, but he blames it on fat, flour, cereal, and a sedentary lifestyle. We should focus our energy on educating the public about sensible eating and physical activity, he suggests, while "allowing Americans to enjoy the simple pleasure of a Coca-Cola."

The Coca-Cola Company has recently formed a partnership with the American Academy of Family Physicians to promote "healthier, active lifestyles" that *include* sweetened beverages; the move is akin to Fredrick Stare's midcentury affiliation with the sugar industry. To make it "easier" to make "positive changes," according to its print ads, the company introduced "90-calorie, portion-control mini-cans" of Coke and Sprite in the New York City and Washington, DC, metro markets in late fall of 2009, with a nationwide rollout to follow, because "achieving a balanced diet . . . doesn't mean you have to sacrifice everything you enjoy." At $7\frac{1}{2}$ ounces, with an image of the original, 6-ounce bottle on the can, it is, at least, a start. Coca-Cola has acknowledged the problem, and even if the company doesn't take responsibility for its role in increasing obesity, it does admit that diet may be a contributing factor, and that something has to change.

THE SINFUL TAX

Coca-Cola, in conjunction with others in the soft drink industry, is also reaching out to consumers to fight the tax. A recent television commercial

211

depicts a well-dressed, thin woman anxiously and sadly explaining that taxing soda would present a hardship for her family that "they" (presumably elitist health nuts) just don't understand. In other words, working-class Americans would be penalized, which is a weak line of self-serving logic, and one that ignores all of the negative implications of making sweetened sodas, low-priced thanks to corn subsidies, among the cheapest products on the market. The slim, middle-class woman isn't concerned about the high costs of produce, whole grains, dairy products, and seafood; she is just upset that the cost of liquid candy, one of the least-expensive items in her shopping cart, might increase.

Is taxing a product that can harm but not help the ethical choice? And where do we draw the line? It may seem unfair that calorically sweetened beverages are being singled out in a supermarket crowded with unhealthy competition, and perhaps it is. But the government owes it to the public to take measures to reverse the high rates of overweight and obesity. And sodas—which, by sheer caloric volume and complete lack of nutritive value, are the worst offenders—seem as good a place to start as any.

26

THE 100-YEAR DIET

CLEMENTINE PADDLEFORD SOUNDS LIKE THE NAME OF A HEROINE IN A CHILDREN'S
book, and indeed, it seemed fitting for a journalist from Kansas who took
her cat to the office and traveled more than 50,000 miles a year by train,
automobile, commercial airplane, and mule; on foot; and even by piloting
her own small Piper Cub in search of material for her columns. Paddleford's beat for *This Week,* the Sunday supplement magazine for the *New
York Herald Tribune* in the mid-20th century, was the kitchens of unknown
but extraordinary regional American home cooks. Crab timbale in New
Orleans, "topped with chives or—feeling rich—a spoonful of caviar." Fried
turkey with corn on the cob and snap beans in Rehoboth Beach, Delaware.
Lobster and Indian pudding in Cohasset, Massachusetts. Danish fried
pancakes called Ebleskivers in Racine, Wisconsin. Blackfish chowder in
Newport, Rhode Island. These were the enticing dishes that motivated her
to crisscross the continent. At a late-November 1950 luncheon table set up
under shade trees at Almaden Vineyard in northern California, she wrote
about being served a "medley of greens" dressed with a vinaigrette that
was "the quintessence of simplicity, made with California olive oil, red
wine and tarragon vinegars," followed by ham from "hogs raised right
here," freshly picked green beans sprinkled with cheese and browned in
the oven, turkey with "slivers of truffles inserted just under the skin," and
fresh freestone peach halves peeled and sprinkled with cognac for dessert.
(She suggests that champagne would also work nicely in place of the
cognac.)

In 1949, Paddleford told a writer for the *Saturday Evening Post*: "We
all have hometown appetites. Every other person is a bundle of longing

213

for the simplicities of good taste once enjoyed on the farm or in the hometown they left behind." And so in 1948 America, when the country was just about to experience the opening of fast food outlets at every highway exit and on street corners in every town, Clem, as her friends called her, was on a quest for the best local recipes she could find to share with "every *other* person"—her readers, those who cared about the quality of their food.

One year after beginning her culinary excursions, she wrote, "If there is an American culture—some say there isn't—surely it is coming in by way of the kitchen door." And though she adds that women are "no longer suspicious" when it comes to "frozen foods, canned goods, and ready-mixes," they were, nevertheless, "taking pride in knowing how to cook." And bake. "Diets come and diets go," she notes, "but pie leads on. [It is] our greatest culinary achievement."

Ever since food processing began in the mid-19th century, there have been contradictions and controversies about how America eats (which was the title of Paddleford's column) and how America *should* eat. Our food may be created from a mix or from scratch, be presented in barely recognizable parts or "whole," and be up-sized or downsized, but rarely is it just right. The paradoxes can be seen in Paddleford's praising both the great culinary achievements of regional American cooks and their prowess with can openers in the same paragraph. ("How does America eat? She eats in a hurry," using "shortcuts" and "instant everything" she mentions in another column.) We are a large and diverse country. While some readers experimented with the recipes Paddleford provided, visiting their local fishmongers to select just the right fillets to use in a flavorful San Francisco cioppino for example, others simply executed them as best they could using the frozen, canned, and processed goods available at their local supermarkets. Socioeconomic status, educational level, ethnicity, time, talent, and geography all play parts in how we eat as a nation. And we display conflicting habits when it comes to food. In 1910, a wealthy patron who was carefully recording every calorie eaten in a sparse, vegetarian, alcohol-free dinner at John Harvey Kellogg's San might in the following week be dining on roast beef, potatoes lyonnaise, charlotte russe, imported cheeses, and wine at Delmonico's elegant Fifth Avenue restaurant in New York City.

As a nation, we've been on a dietary seesaw for a long time, in part because diets do come and go, but our love affair with pie remains constant. In a 2008 Nielsen survey, 81 percent of Americans believed that overweight is a direct result of eating too much and moving too little. A positive development is that fewer than 10 percent planned to cut back by following a fad diet or by joining Weight Watchers; instead, their strategy is to make real, sustainable dietary changes such as eating less fat and sugar and eating smaller portions. There is a lot of perceived room for improvement—only 14 percent of those polled rated their diets as "healthy." Best-selling book franchises such as David Zinczenko and Matt Goulding's *Eat This, Not That!* and Mehmet Oz and Michael Roizen's *You* series promote the idea that small, consistent, incremental changes will yield the best results over the long haul, a weight-loss model that is growing in popularity. It's easier, after all, to choose a less-fattening hamburger than to swear off hamburgers entirely. There are still fad diets out there, to be sure, but there are fewer of them than in previous decades, and some of the more sensible, nutritionally sound programs appear to be catching on. As Sherlock Holmes said to Dr. Watson in *The Sign of the Four,* "when you have eliminated the impossible, whatever remains, *however improbable,* must be the truth." And the truth is that the vast majority of us weigh too much as a result of our unhealthy diets and lack of exercise. That bit of information was published for the first time in 1727 in London, when it was based entirely on observation. It appears to be immutable.

A lot of other valuable information about the way we eat is starting to get attention. Harvey Wiley, who spent his career fighting for pure, wholesome food that was priced high enough to adequately support the farmers who produced it, believed "Any man who adds . . . to the food he sells [an additive] which renders it dangerous strikes at the very existence of the human race, because a man is what he eats, and if you change his food you change the man." He would have been one of journalist and activist Eric Schlosser's biggest fans. When Schlosser's *Fast Food Nation: The Dark Side of the All-American Meal* was published in 2001, its impact on public opinion was on a scale similar to that exerted by Upton Sinclair's 1906 exposé of the meatpacking industry, *The Jungle*. Schlosser's book also had a tremendous influence on McDonald's and many other fast food chains, whose menus now include more salads and other lower-calorie, healthier alternatives.

America has produced some excellent and inspirational food writers—A. J. Liebling, Waverly Root, and M. F. K. Fisher wrote eloquently about the pleasures of dining well. But their compelling prose was inspired by eating in Italy and France. (Even Harvey Wiley's introduction to Mildred Maddocks Bentley's 1914 *Pure Food Cook Book* begins in Burgundy, where he marvels at the simple goodness of the beautifully prepared, local, home-cooked foods.) Margaret and Ancel Keys wrote and spoke about the joys and health benefits of eating fresh, local Mediterranean foods in the 1950s. In the 1970s, Alice Waters brought local back home. This was a "new" type of cuisine—a passion for the freshest, pesticide-free produce picked the day you cooked it, as if you were on an 18th-century farm—or in the French or Italian countryside. (Or, midcentury, lunching with Clem at Almaden Vineyard in northern California.) Waters's philosophy treated farmers, as well as farm animals, with respect. She emphasized that exquisite ingredients should be prepared simply in order to showcase their incredible natural flavors and keep their nutritive benefits intact. All of this was accomplished at Chez Panisse, the Berkeley, California, restaurant that is as popular as ever and whose kitchen has produced some of the brightest talents on the American culinary scene.

The great popularity of cooking shows has transformed many chefs into celebrities in their own rights. In fact, in recent years, the career choice of chef no longer conjures up an image of difficult, blue-collar toil, but rather is aspired to by many who believe that going to culinary school will someday turn them into toque-wearing rock stars. Small farming, too, has taken on a kind of rustic chic, as local food enthusiasts eagerly seek out their goods and restaurants proudly list the family farms that supply their kitchens on their seasonal menus.

Valuing the quality and origin of our food, as Sylvester Graham urged us to do when he stipulated that processing wheat could be a dangerous thing, was strongly reinforced in the last decade, when writers like Michael Pollan, Mark Bittman, and Barbara Kingsolver explained why we Americans should be skeptical about processed foods and factory farms and either support small, organic, local farmers or grow and raise the food ourselves for the sake of our health and the health of the planet. Their books became bestsellers that Graham and Kellogg would have loved.

John Mackey's 1,100-square-foot Whole Foods Market, a smash hit when he opened it in Austin, Texas, in 1980, became a national chain by the mid-1990s. Shopping for organic (and often local) produce outside of farmers' markets or in wintertime had never been easier (at least in middle-class neighborhoods), and his success has led most supermarkets and discounters to now stock at least some organic items. Sales of UPC-coded organic foods increased by 132 percent between 2004 and 2008, a figure that would surely be greater if sales by merchants at the farmers' markets that have sprung up all over the country could be captured. Organic food has become so mainstream that the "secret ingredient" of the first Iron Chef competition televised in 2010 was anything the chefs chose to harvest from the organic garden on the White House lawn. "Organics are on fire, with billions in sales" the latest Nielsen survey reports. The more mainstream whole and organic foods become, the better, not only because we will be consuming fewer pesticides, but also because the more we think about what we eat, the less likely we are to eat too much.

It may seem as though we have come full circle, or perhaps that we haven't traveled at all. But it's undeniable that in America today, there are vocal and articulate leaders with large followings who demand a purer food supply—a plant-based diet of pesticide- and additive-free fruits, vegetables, and whole grains. ("The whiter the bread, the sooner you'll be dead," Michael Pollan exclaims in *Food Rules: An Eater's Manual*. Sylvester Graham couldn't have said it better.) College students are eating less meat, and many young people are becoming vegetarian or vegan, with the result that Graham-style menus are prevalent in their campus dining halls. Large industrial agribusinesses demonize this movement as (what else?) elitist, claiming that "organic" is just another word for expensive—kind of like the food processors who once opposed Graham, Wiley, and their followers. As diverse ethnic groups continue to immigrate to the United States and open restaurants across the country, culinary options will continue to expand for adventurous diners. But those newly arrived immigrants are still being forced into a homogenized, Americanized way of eating, only now it is at the urging of value-priced fast food chains rather than of patriotic home economists. Delmonico's in New York City closed in 1923, a victim of Prohibition and changing tastes, according to the *New York Times*. But the New Orleans branch of the popular eatery, which opened in 1895, is now owned by celebrity chef Emeril Lagasse. And it is thriving. It may seem that the more things change ("I'll have the sushi"), the more they stay the same ("I'll have the pie"). Except, of course, 100 years ago the industrialization of our food supply was in its infancy, and most Americans didn't need to lose weight.

Raising awareness about what we eat and why, and about how to do better, is our best opportunity to reverse the trend. Food Network shows, culinary blogs, food magazines, food books, food newspaper coverage, and even the First Lady's efforts—we have never had so much easily accessible, high-quality information about our food supply's products and processes. This is not irrational optimism; important steps are being taken at both the national and the local levels to reduce obesity and improve the quality of our diets. For example, the pledges made by Coca-Cola and Pepsi-Cola to the William J. Clinton Foundation and American Heart Association's anti-childhood-obesity alliance to eliminate sweetened sodas from school vending machines have gone into effect. Chain restaurants in New York City now must, by law, post calorie counts on menus; so, too, must concession stands at the movies, and similar laws are being passed in many other cities and towns as well. New York City schools no longer allow bake sales during class hours, which may seem like a minor measure, but it is indicative of a very different way of thinking about pie. Many cities and counties ban their restaurants from cooking with trans fats, and on January 2, 2010, California became the first state to do so. (Also known as partially hydrogenated cooking oils, trans fats decrease HDL, or "good" cholesterol, and increase LDL, or "bad" cholesterol. Ancel Keys's theory that cholesterol caused heart disease, as it turns out, was only partially right.) These changes will be incorporated into the ways that many Americans choose what to eat, both inside and outside the home.

In 1909, the *Washington Post* printed a poem called "Hopeless Case." The neighbor of the poem's narrator is trying to lose weight, but is going about it, the poet seems certain, in the wrong way. This is the last stanza:

> *Never quiet, has to diet.*
> *Starves herself to death.*
> *With her banting. Always panting. Running out of breath.*
> *She will shortly be more portly*
> *Or I'll eat my hat.*
> *Nothing to it! I'd not do it.*
> *Even were I fat.*

During World War II (and prior to the widespread adoption of the Helsinki Declaration*), Ancel Keys studied the effects of semistarvation on healthy male conscientious objectors who had volunteered to help Keys understand the physiological and psychological implications of being undernourished and the best ways to rehabilitate famine victims after the war.

The men were allowed 1,600 calories a day, or about half of what they required to maintain their very active lifestyles. They lost weight, and they also suffered from depression and displayed neurotic and psychotic behavior. After a period of controlled refeeding, they were allowed to eat whatever they desired and ended up an average of 5 percent heavier than they had been when they joined the study.

Starvation diets are dangerous and ineffective, and even some of Keys's extremely dedicated and closely watched volunteers cheated. Many fad diets allow fewer calories than Keys allowed his subjects. And they all guarantee that shortly, you'll be more portly.

---

* This code for conducting ethical human research was first adopted in 1964 in Helsinki, Finland, and has been revised numerous times since.

CONCLUSION
THE OBESITY TRIANGLE

AN INFECTIOUS DISEASE LIKE THE FLU NEEDS THREE THINGS TO BECOME AN epidemic: an external agent (the virus), a host (you or me), and an environment eager to connect us (the guy with a cough on your flight or the sneezing woman next to you in the elevator). This is called an epidemiological triad.

A similar triad has been applied to obesity. The external agent includes the separate elements of increased portion sizes, technologically driven lifestyle changes, and the 24/7 availability of fast and convenience foods. As hosts, in this case we do more than just breathe in when we're in the wrong place at the wrong time. Lack of education about good nutrition, health-positive behaviors and attitudes, and human physiology; lack of adequate exercise; and lack of a sense of responsibility and of forethought about health all contribute to the epidemic. The environmental factors stem from the institutionalized, systematic support of the problem—including political, economic, and social influences. And like a virus, obesity can be "caught," because we tend to mirror the activities of those around us.

Nicholas Christakis, MD, PhD, a physician and sociologist who teaches at Harvard, and James Fowler, PhD, a political scientist at the University of California at San Diego, analyzed Framingham Heart Study data to evaluate how an interconnected social network of 12,067 people influenced each other over a span of 32 years. Because body mass index data were available for all the subjects, this was an ideal way to track the social components of weight. The results were published in the July 26, 2007, issue of the *New England Journal of Medicine.* Christakis and Fowler determined that a person's chance of becoming obese increased by 57 percent if a friend became obese during the same time period. If an adult sibling became obese, the chance increased by 40 percent; if a spouse became obese, the likelihood increased by 37 percent. Amazingly, there appeared to be three degrees of separation—the chance of a person becoming obese increased by 20 percent if a friend of a friend became obese, even if the friend did not. And yet, neighbors who were not friends had no influence on weight. Christakis and Fowler concluded, "Obesity appears to spread through social ties."

In other words, it's contagious.

TEACH YOUR CHILDREN / FEED THEM ON YOUR DREAMS

Although it has often been said that "everyone knows" how to eat right and how to lose weight, that isn't true. We have been doing a poor job of educating our children about how to make good nutritional decisions at home and at school, and hopefully that is about to change. Making kids aware of the elements of an optimal diet and the negative results of a bad one is the first line of defense, and the best. Class trips to a local supermarket that include instruction about what to purchase and what to avoid should begin in the third grade.

So should instruction on basic cooking skills, which has disappeared from most public school classrooms. If we teach children how to prepare salads, vegetables, and simple, nutritious meals during grade school, everyone *will* know what to eat and how to cook it. This is every bit as important to our children's futures as science and mathematics are. It also can be a terrific way to teach those subjects.

Children should also learn about the origins of the foods on their plates—how they got from the farms to the tables. They should be taught how to plant seeds, help them grow, and reap the fruits of their labor. And we should instruct them in the fundamentals of proper food handling, including how to recognize what is safe for them to eat. In 2009, severe food-related illnesses and deaths resulted from consuming peanut butter,

221

raw Toll House cookie dough, and hamburger. The system put in place to protect us from such harm is failing badly when Jeffrey Bender, DVM, a veterinarian and food safety expert who developed methods for tracing *Escherichia coli* contamination, is quoted in the *New York Times* as saying: "Ground beef is not a completely safe product."

If food appears to be impossibly cheap, there is always a reason. Cargill's American Chef's Selection Angus Beef Patties, the hamburger infected with *E. coli* that paralyzed a 22-year-old children's dance instructor in 2009, contained ground beef from Nebraska, Texas, South Dakota, and Uruguay, some of which had been treated with ammonia to reduce the numbers of the bacteria to undetectable levels. Shipping improperly treated and inspected ground beef and fat from numerous locations to be processed with bread crumb fillers and shipped again in American Chef's Selection packages saved Cargill 30 cents a pound. Some of those "savings" were passed on to the young dancer.

While companies like Cargill make large profits,* we all pay a huge price for inexpensive foods in the forms of subsidies, fossil fuel use, medical bills, and personal tragedy. The high price of cheap food permeates all of our lives. "Why so cheap?" is as valid a question as "Why so expensive?"

AN EXCELLENT PLACE TO START

Writer and agrarian Wendell Berry, who has been trying hard to educate us about how to eat and live well for more than 40 years, once eloquently described a New England farm in the first half of the 20th century as modest but successful because "its needs were kept within the limits of its resources."

I can't imagine a better way to frame a diet, or a life, for the next 100 years.

---

* Cargill is the largest privately owned business in America, with $116.6 billion in 2008 revenues.

BIBLIOGRAPHY

Agatston, Arthur. *The South Beach Diet.* Emmaus, PA: Rodale, 2003.

Alexander, Kelly, and Cynthia Harris. *Hometown Appetites.* New York: Gotham Books, 2008.

Allport, Susan. *The Queen of Fats.* Berkeley, CA: University of California Press, 2006.

Atkins, Robert C. *Dr. Atkins' Diet Revolution: The High Calorie Way to Stay Thin Forever.* New York: D. McKay, 1972.

———. *Dr. Atkins' New Diet Revolution.* New York: Avon Books, 2002.

Bacon, Linda. *Health at Every Size: The Surprising Truth about Your Weight.* Dallas: Benbella Books, 2008.

Bennett, William, and Joel Gurin. *Dieter's Dilemma: Eating Less and Weighing More.* New York: Basic Books, 1982.

Berry, Wendell. "Energy in Agriculture." In *Bringing It to the Table: On Farming and Food*, 57–65. Berkeley, CA: Counterpoint, 2009.

Bittman, Mark. *Food Matters.* New York: Simon and Schuster, 2009.

Brody, Jane. *Jane Brody's Nutrition Book.* New York: Norton, 1981.

Bruch, Hilde. "Body Image and Self-Awareness." In *Food and Culture*, edited by Carole Counihan and Penny Van Esterik, 211–25. New York: Routledge, 1997.

Campos, Paul. *The Obesity Myth.* New York: Gotham Books, 2004.

Carson, Gerald. *Cornflake Crusade.* New York: Rinehart, 1957.

Cohen, Rich. *Sweet and Low: A Family Story.* New York: Farrar, Straus and Giroux, 2006.

Critser, Greg. *Fat Land: How Americans Became the Fattest People in the World.* Boston: Houghton Mifflin, 2003.

De Groot, Roy Andries. *How I Reduced with the New Rockefeller Diet: Part 1. The Rockefeller Diet. Part 2. The Diet for Gourmets.* New York: Horizon Press, 1956.

———. *Feasts for All Seasons.* New York: Knopf, 1966.

Delpeuch, Francis, Bernard Maire, Emmanuel Monnier, and Michelle Holdsworth. *Globesity: A Planet Out of Control?* Sterling, VA: Earthscan, 2009.

Donaldson, Blake F. *Strong Medicine.* New York: Doubleday, 1962.

Donnelly, Antoinette. *How to Reduce: New Waistlines for Old.* New York: D. Appleton, 1920.

Farmer, Fannie Merritt. *The Original Boston Cooking-School Cook Book.* Westport, CT: Hugh Lauter Levin Associates, 1996.

Finkelstein, Eric A., and Laurie Zuckerman. *The Fattening of America.* Hoboken, NJ: Wiley, 2008.

Fiore, Evelyn L., ed. *The Low Carbohydrate Diet: The Widely Circulated Diet Usually Called "the Air Force Diet," Now for the First Time with Complete*

List of Carbohydrate and Calorie Content of All Common Foods. New York: Nelson, 1965.

Gratzer, Walter. *Terrors of the Table: The Curious History of Nutrition.* Oxford, England: Oxford University Press, 2005.

Grover, Kathryn, ed. *Fitness in American Culture.* Amherst, MA: University of Massachusetts Press, 1989.

Hauser, Bengamin Gayelord. *Look Younger, Live Longer.* New York: Farrar, Straus, 1951.

Heimann, Jim, ed. *All-American Ads of the '30s.* Cologne, Germany: Taschen, 2003.

Hu, Frank B., ed. *Obesity Epidemiology.* New York: Oxford University Press, 2008.

Hurst, Fannie. *Anatomy of Me: A Wonderer in Search of Herself.* Garden City, NY: Doubleday, 1958.

———. *No Food with My Meals.* New York: Harper and Brothers, 1935.

Jolliffe, Norman. *Reduce and Stay Reduced.* New York: Simon and Schuster, 1952.

Kellogg, John Harvey. *The Battle Creek Sanitarium Diet List.* Battle Creek, MI: Modern Medicine, 1909.

———. *The Battle Creek Sanitarium System: History, Organization, Methods.* Battle Creek, MI: Gage Printing, 1908.

Kessler, David A. *The End of Overeating: Taking Control of the Insatiable American Appetite.* New York: Rodale, 2009.

Keys, Ancel. *The Biology of Human Starvation.* Minneapolis: University of Minnesota Press, 1950.

Keys, Ancel and Margaret. *Eat Well and Stay Well.* Garden City, NY: Doubleday, 1959.

———. *How to Eat Well and Stay Well the Mediterranean Way.* Garden City, NY: Doubleday, 1975.

Keys, Margaret and Ancel. *The Benevolent Bean.* Garden City, NY: Doubleday, 1967.

Kingsolver, Barbara. *Animal, Vegetable, Miracle: A Year of Food.* New York: HarperCollins, 2007.

Koten, Bernard. *The Low-Calory Cookbook.* New York: Random House, 1951.

Lehrer, Jonah. *How We Decide.* New York: Houghton Mifflin Harcourt, 2009.

Levenstein, Harvey. *Paradox of Plenty: A Social History of Eating in Modern America.* Berkeley, CA: University of California Press, 2003.

———. *Revolution at the Table: The Transformation of the American Diet.* Berkeley, CA: University of California Press, 2003.

Lowe, Margaret A. "From Robust Appetites to Counting Calories: The Emergence of Dieting among Smith College Students in the 1920s." In *Women and Health in America,* 2nd ed., edited by Judith Walzer Leavitt, 172–89. Madison, WI: University of Wisconsin Press, 1995.

Malmberg, Carl. *Diet and Die.* New York: Hillman-Curl, 1935.

Mazel, Judy, with Susan Shultz. *The Beverly Hills Diet.* New York: Macmillan, 1981.

Mazel, Judy, and Michael Wyatt. *The New Beverly Hills Diet: The Latest Weight-Loss Research That Explains a Conscious Food-Combining Program for Life-Long Slimhood.* Deerfield Beach, FL: Health Communications, 1996.

McClellan, Walter S., and Eugene F. Du Bois. "Clinical Calorimetry. XLV. Prolonged Meat Diets with a Study of Kidney Function and Ketosis." *Journal of Biological Chemistry* 87 (1930): 651–68. http://www.jbc.org/cgi/reprint/87/3/651.pdf.

Mintz, Sidney W. *Sweetness and Power.* New York: Penguin Books, 1986.

Montagné, Prosper. *Larousse Gastronomique.* New York: Crown, 1961.

Nestle, Marion. *Food Politics: How the Food Industry Influences Nutrition and Health.* Berkeley, CA: University of California Press, 2002.

Nidetch, Jean, with Joan Rattner Heilman. *The Story of Weight Watchers.* New York: W/W TwentyFirst, 1970.

Nissenbaum, Stephen. *Sex, Diet, and Debility in Jacksonian America: Sylvester Graham and Health Reform.* Westport, CT: Greenwood Press, 1980.

Ornish, Dean. *Eat More, Weigh Less.* New York: HarperCollins, 1993.

Paddleford, Clementine. *How America Eats.* New York: Charles Scribner's Sons, 1960.

Pálsson, Gísli. *Travelling Passions: The Hidden Life of Vilhjalmur Stefansson.* Edited by Keneva Kunz. Hanover, NH: Dartmouth College Press, 2005.

Peters, Lulu Hunt. *Diet and Health, with Key to the Calories.* Chicago: Reilly and Lee, 1918. http://www.gutenberg.org/etext/15069.

Pollan, Michael. *In Defense of Food: An Eater's Manifesto.* New York: Penguin, 2008.

———. *Food Rules: An Eater's Manual.* New York: Penguin, 2009.

Popkin, Barry. *The World Is Fat: The Fads, Trends, Policies, and Products That Are Fattening the Human Race.* New York: Avery, 2009.

Pritikin, Nathan. *The Pritikin Permanent Weight-Loss Manual.* New York: Grosset and Dunlap, 1981.

Pritikin, Robert. *The Pritikin Weight Loss Breakthrough.* New York: Dutton, 1998.

Rasenberger, Jim. *America, 1908.* New York: Scribner, 2007.

Roizen, Michael F., and Mehmet Oz. *You, On a Diet.* New York: Free Press, 2006.

Rombauer, Irma S. *The Joy of Cooking: A Facsimile of the First Edition 1931.* New York: Scribner, 1998.

Ross, Bruce. "Fat or Fiction." In *The Obesity Epidemic: Science, Morality and Ideology,* edited by Michael Gard and Jan Wright, 86–106. New York: Routledge, 2005.

Schwartz, Hillel. *Never Satisfied: A Cultural History of Diets, Fantasies, and Fat.* New York: Free Press, 1986.

Seid, Roberta Pollack. *Never Too Thin: Why Women Are at War with Their Bodies.* New York: Prentice Hall Press, 1989.

Standage, Tom. *A History of the World in 6 Glasses.* New York: Walker, 2005.

Stanley, Autumn. *Mothers and Daughters of Invention.* New Brunswick, NJ: Rutgers University Press, 1995.

Stearns, Peter N. *Fat History: Bodies and Beauty in the Modern West.* New York: New York University Press, 1997.

Stefansson, Vilhjalmur. *The Fat of the Land.* New York: Macmillan, 1956.

———. *The Friendly Arctic.* New York: Macmillan, 1943.

———. *Not by Bread Alone.* New York: Macmillan, 1946.

Steward, H. Leighton, Morrison C. Bethea, Samuel S. Andrews, and Luis A. Balart. *Sugar Busters!* New York: Ballantine, 1998.

Taller, Herman. *Calories Don't Count.* New York: Simon and Schuster, 1961.

Tarnower, Herman, and Samm Sinclair Baker. *The Complete Scarsdale Medical Diet Plus Dr. Tarnower's Lifetime Keep-Slim Program.* New York: Rawson, Wade, 1978.

Taubes, Gary. *Good Calories, Bad Calories: Fats, Carbs, and the Controversial Science of Diet and Health.* New York: Anchor Books, 2008.

Thompson, Vance. *Eat and Grow Thin: The Mahdah Menus.* New York: E. P. Dutton, 1914.

Trilling, Diana. *Mrs. Harris: The Death of the Scarsdale Diet Doctor.* New York: Harcourt Brace Jovanovich, 1981.

Whelan, Elizabeth M., and Fredrick J. Stare. *Panic in the Pantry.* New York: Atheneum, 1975.

Wiley, Harvey. *An Autobiography.* Indianapolis: Bobbs-Merrill, 1930.

ENDNOTES

Introduction

p. ix **a popular trick** "In the Effort to be Angular the Fat Woman Terrifies Her Thin Sister; Physician Points Out the Dangers in Various Systems Followed in Attempt to Reduce Flesh. Banting Is the Silliest Idea We Have, He Thinks," *New York Times*, August 11, 1907.

p. ix *Letter on Corpulence* William Banting, *Letter on Corpulence, Addressed to the Public* (London: Harrison, 1863). The third edition is available at http://www.archive.org/details/letteroncorpulen00bant.

p. ix **America's first diet book** However, it was not Britain's first monograph on the topic, which is believed to have been Thomas Short's *A Discourse Concerning the Causes and Effects of Corpulency: Together with the Method for Its Prevention and Cure*, published in London in 1727 by J. Roberts.

p. ix **he felt obligated to share Dr. Harvey's knowledge with the world** In 1872, William Harvey published *On Corpulence in Relation to Disease: With Some Remarks on Diet* (London: Henry Renshaw), and by doing so he gave scientific endorsement to Banting's claims. Harvey began this treatise with Hippocrates' words: "Corpulence is not only a disease itself, but the harbinger of others."

p. x **It was well received** "How to Get Thin," *New York Times*, October 14, 1883.

p. x **fat in foods (including bacon) actually made pounds disappear** "Fat as a Cure of Obesity," *New York Times*, May 2, 1884.

p. xii **the Sinner's Table** "The Solving of the Meat Problem: What Has Been Accomplished at the Battle Creek Sanitarium During the Past Thirty-Seven Years," *Chicago Daily Tribune*, June 5, 1902, p. 7. Retrieved January 18, 2010, from ProQuest Historical Newspapers Chicago Tribune (1849–1986). (Document ID: 408547801).

Chapter 1

p. 3 **debauchery-filled lifestyle and diet could lead to illness and death** Stephen Nissenbaum, *Sex, Diet, and Debility in Jacksonian America: Sylvester Graham and Health Reform* (Westport, CT: Greenwood Press, 1980), 6–91; and Hillel Schwartz, *Never Satisfied: A Cultural History of Diets, Fantasies, and Fat* (New York: Free Press, 1986).

p. 3 **citing as evidence** Sylvester Graham, "A Lecture on Epidemic Diseases Generally, and Particularly the Spasmodic Cholera" (lecture, New York, March 1832).

p. 4 **As correspondent J. M. Bishop stated** J. M. Bishop, "How to Live Economically," *New York Times*, September 26, 1898. What begins as an argument for meatless meals as an economical way to control the family food budget ends with the widespread belief of the day—eating animal protein leads to immorality.

p. 4 **Treat your stomach like a well governed child** Sylvester Graham, introduction to *Discourses on a Sober and Temperate Life*, by Luigi Cornaro (London: Benjamin White, 1823).

p. 4 **meant to be consumed only after becoming stale** Sylvester Graham, *Treatise on Bread, and Bread-Making* (Boston: Light and Stearns, 1837). Graham mentions that if yeast *is* used, bread should not be eaten for at least 24 hours after removal from the oven to allow the alcohol to evaporate.

p. 5 **A typical breakfast** Gerald Carson, *Cornflake Crusade* (New York: Rinehart, 1957), 32. This was breakfast as depicted by the president of Amherst College, the school Sylvester Graham attended in 1823 and 1824.

p. 5 **atonic dyspepsia** Robert Tomes, *The Bazar Book of Decorum* (New York: Harper and Brothers, 1870), 184.

pp. 5–6 **police had to intervene** Graham had recruited the "police" from among his followers; the mayor had told him that there were too many threats for the city to be able to guarantee his protection. They were successful in keeping the butchers and bakers at bay, mainly by heaving shovelfuls of slaked lime over them. Graham escaped unscathed.

p. 6 **Graham board** Williams College and Wesleyan University were the first two to comply.

p. 6 **a feeble condition** R. T. Trall, "Biographical Sketch of Sylvester Graham," *Water-Cure Journal*, November 1851.

pp. 6–7 **the first child to be born** As mentioned in his *New York Times* obituary, published August 9, 1881.

p. 9 **Granose** This was not the first popular cereal product. Dr. James Caleb Jackson, the man who had trained Ellen and James White before they opened their Western Health Reform Institute, had already created a cereal by breaking graham crackers into little pieces, which he named Granula.

p. 9 **Sanitas** There were three separate food-manufacturing offshoots of the San, including the Battle Creek Sanitarium Food Company and the Sanitas Nut Company. In 1906, the Kellogg's Food Company was created to market Kellogg's Corn Flakes; Kellogg's All-Bran was added to the product line in 1908.

p. 10 **came for a rest cure or lifestyle change** "The Solving of the Meat Problem," *Chicago Daily Tribune*, June 5, 1902.

p. 10 **For the woman who was too thin** S. T. Rorer, "The Best Foods for Stout and Thin Women: Domestic Lesson Number 7," *Ladies' Home Journal*, July 1898.

p. 10 **"When a Woman Is Stout"** Virginia Louis Ralston, "When a Woman Is Stout," *Ladies' Home Journal*, February 1902.

p. 10 **a heartbreaking story** "Was Afraid of Anti-Fat," *Washington Post*, November 13, 1899.

p. 11 **Corpulency is the deadliest enemy of the modern daughter of Eve** "Are Society Women Literally Killing Themselves to Keep Thin?" *Chicago Daily Tribune*, June 19, 1910. The anonymous author of this article questions the new trend among the wealthy to "diet" (it's such a new word that it is in quotation marks) to the point of starvation, an early precursor, perhaps, to anorexia.

p. 11 **the first reducing salons opened** Peter Stearns, *Fat History: Bodies and Beauty in the Modern West* (New York: New York University Press, 1997), 21.

p. 11 **The diet is sophisticated and expensive** Vance Thompson, *Eat and Grow Thin: The Mahdah Menus* (New York: E. P. Dutton, 1914). Weight loss for the affluent.

p. 12 **In 1902, Russell Chittenden, a well-respected Yale physiologist and early pioneer in nutrition, invited Fletcher to his university** Burton J. Hendrick, "Some Modern Ideas on Food," *McClure's*, April 1910, 653–69.

p. 13 **the Chittenden standard** The USDA guidelines currently recommend 50 grams of protein daily for a 150-pound male. Eight ounces of lean beef have 64 grams.

p. 13 **The masticating vegetarians won every battle** Hendrick, "Some Modern Ideas."

p. 13 **39 False Food Fads** "False Food Fads Number 39: Physician Gives List of Harmful Diet Doctrines That Have Become Popular," *Washington Post*, April 10, 1910.

p. 13 **I do not believe in fletcherizing. It makes you sick of everything you eat.** "Urges No Breakfast," *Washington Post*, November 25, 1912.

p. 13 **In a single generation the whole social problem would be solved** "Mastication and Social Reform," *Chicago Daily Tribune*, March 19, 1906.

p. 14 **a series of human experiments** As unethical as it may seem today, experimenting on humans was once accepted practice. For example, in 1915 prisoners volunteered (in exchange for parole if they survived) to be fed diets lacking specific nutrients in order to establish a correlation between a deficit of certain B vitamins and pellagra, which was then a dreaded disease often confused with leprosy. In 1943, the Minnesota Experiment used volunteer conscientious objectors to determine the effects of starvation on the human body, with the goal of improving the rehabilitation of famine victims after World War II.

p. 14 **the son of a struggling farmer and strict Calvinist** Information about Harvey Wiley's childhood comes from his charming autobiography, *An Autobiography* (Indianapolis: Bobbs-Merrill, 1930).

p. 15 **Wiley's "Poison Squad"** The *Washington Post* covered the Borax Café in a series of articles beginning in 1902.

p. 16 **"calorie"** "Calorie" is a general term that refers to the energy value of food, based on the fact that 1,000 calories is the amount of energy it takes to heat 1 kilogram of water 1°C. The body burns protein, fat, carbohydrates, and alcohol for energy. Too much of any of them (too many calories) will get stored as fat.

p. 17 ***Boston Cooking-School Cook Book*** Fannie Merritt Farmer, *The Original Boston Cooking-School Cook Book* (Westport, CT: Hugh Lauter Levin Associates, 1996).

p. 17 **a "steam engine in breeches"** Carl Malmberg, *Diet and Die* (New York: Hillman-Curl, 1935), 10.

p. 17 **Dietetics has at long last come to be a science** John Harvey Kellogg, *The Battle Creek Sanitarium Diet List* (Battle Creek, MI: Modern Medicine, 1909).

Chapter 2

p. 18 **If an Italian family could find imported olive oil** Harvey Levenstein, *Revolution at the Table* (Berkeley, CA: University of California Press, 2003), 103.

p. 19 **While her classmates were learning to embroider a tablecloth or frost a cake** *History of Milford* (Milford, ME: Milford Bicentennial Committee, 1976).

p. 20 **I almost hate my husband when I think how long he kept me under that delusion** Lulu Hunt Peters, *Diet and Health, with Key to the Calories* (Chicago: Reilly and Lee, 1918), 18–9.

p. 20 ***Now fat individuals have always been considered a joke*** Ibid., 13.

p. 21 **If democracy is worth anything** "Hoover Says Victory Depends Upon Food," *Washington Post*, June 10, 1917.

p. 21 **All fed!** "All Fed, Says Hoover," *Washington Post*, August 24, 1918.

p. 22 **[Most disease] can be prevented** Lulu Hunt Peters, "Diet and Health," *Los Angeles Times*, April 25, 1922.

p. 23 **he surprised the town by secretly marrying** "Dr. W.A. Evans' Secret Out," *Chicago Daily Tribune*, November 21, 1907.

p. 23 **Eat less.** W. A. Evans, "How to Keep Well," March 9, 1925.

p. 24 **obesity is a serious hindrance to the enjoyment and comfort of life** Evans, "How to Keep Well," November 4, 1911.

p. 24 **In 1912, he printed some unwieldy calorie and protein charts** Evans, "How to Keep Well," February 19, 1912.

p. 24 **On Christmas Eve of 1913** Evans, "How to Keep Well," December 24, 1913.

p. 24 **In April of 1915, he printed up-to-date charts** Evans, "How to Keep Well," April 30, 1915.

p. 25 **In 1931, Evans retracted the idea that weight should increase with age** Evans, "How to Keep Well," September 14, 1931.

p. 25 **by 1925 the congenial doctor had become cruel** Evans, "How to Keep Well," March 9, 1925.

p. 25 **In the mid-1920s, Evans, like Peters, believed that most Americans weighed too much** Evans, "How to Keep Well," February 11, 1925.

p. 25 ***A good appetite. There you are, fat folks*** William Brady, "Health Talks," *Atlanta Constitution*, January 14, 1925.

p. 26 **How anyone could want to be anything but thin was beyond my comprehension** Lulu Hunt Peters, "Diet and Health," *Los Angeles Times,* May 29, 1922.

p. 26 **The 1883 class of men entering Yale averaged about 5 feet 8 inches and weighed 138 pounds** Hillel Schwartz, *Never Satisfied: A Cultural History of Diets, Fantasies, and Fat* (New York: Free Press, 1986), 157.

p. 26   **Young women in the Midwest averaged 5 feet 3 inches and 114 pounds in 1893**   Ibid.

p. 27   **In 1928, Americans were eating 5 percent *fewer* calories per capita than they had in 1890**   Levenstein, *Revolution at the Table*, 194.

p. 27   **Science has determined the correct weight for everyone, according to height and age and sex**   Detecto Scale Company, *Los Angeles Times*, June 18, 1929, A3 (advertisement).

p. 27   **how the Continental Scale Company brochure put it**   Schwartz, *Never Satisfied*, 170.

p. 27   **You could "safeguard your health" for $12.95 or less, or 50 cents a week, no money down**   Detecto Scale Company, *Los Angeles Times*, February 10, 1929, 2 (advertisement).

p. 28   **It seems as though just about everyone used penny scales, whether they owned bathroom scales or not**   "Fat Women Busy Reducing, Thin Ones Adding Weight," *New York Times*, July 26, 1925.

p. 28   **dropping 500 million pennies into the slots**   "Penny Scales Make Millions," *New York Times*, July 10, 1927.

p. 28   **The wife of the distributor of Roberts Weight-O-Health weighing machines**   "Pennies, Pennies, Pennies, Thirty Thousand of Them," *Los Angeles Times*, February 5, 1928.

p. 28   **If you were too thin, you could drink the "bodybuilder" called Todd's Tonic**   Todd's Tonic, *Washington Post*, February 12, 1926, 8 (advertisement).

p. 29   **the *New York Times* suggested that it was so comfortable**   "Garments for Reducing," *New York Times*, August 17, 1924.

p. 29   **Woman's figure is the exclamation point of the world!**   *Vogue*, January 1, 1923.

p. 29   **A former American Medical Association president, Woods Hutchinson, MD**   Roberta Pollack Seid, *Never Too Thin: Why Women Are at War with Their Bodies* (New York: Prentice Hall, 1989), 99.

p. 30   **In 1924, three students coauthored a letter to the editor of the *Smith College Weekly***   Margaret A. Lowe, "From Robust Appetites to Calorie Counting: The Emergence of Dieting Among Smith College Students in the 1920s," in *Women and Health in America*, 2nd ed., ed. Judith Walzer Leavitt (Madison, WI: University of Wisconsin Press, 1995), 173.

p. 30   **an automobile race that began in Times Square and ended in Paris by way of the frozen Bering Strait**   Jim Rasenberger describes this in detail in *America, 1908: The Dawn of Flight, the Race to the Pole, the Invention of the Model T, and the Making of a Modern Nation* (New York: Scribner, 2007).

p. 30   **It looked like a convention of circus heavyweights**   "Chicago Conducting an Official Weight Reducing Class," *New York Tribune*, May 9, 1920.

p. 31   **the national feminine cry is not votes for women—but fatless figures for women**   Antoinette Donnelly, *How to Reduce: New Waistlines for Old* (New York: D. Appleton, 1920), vii.

p. 31   **The Robertson–Donnelly stunt was scheduled to last 7 weeks**   The *Chicago Daily Tribune* follows it on a regular basis from beginning to end. See, in particular, April 24, April 28, May 9, and May 23.

p. 33   **police had to be called in to prevent a riot**   "Fat New Yorkers in Race to Reduce," *Chicago Daily Tribune*, October 23, 1921.

p. 34   **intoxication—if not too advanced a stage—counts not at all against one**   *Vogue*, January 1, 1923.

p. 34   **Archived letters from Smith women prior to 1920 often mentioned the need to gain weight, and a lot of it**   Lowe, "From Robust Appetites to Calorie Counting," 37.

p. 34   **Lulu Hunt Peters was the voice of reason**   Lulu Hunt Peters, "Diet and Health," *Los Angeles Times*, January 21, 1925.

p 34   **In the same year Peters proposed an obesity tax**   "Reduce or Pay Tax. Woman Physician's Plan for Fat Folk," *Chicago Daily Tribune*, April 28, 1925.

p. 35   **In 1930, historian Eunice Fuller Barnard wrote**   Eunice Fuller Barnard, "In Food, Also, a New Fashion Is Here," *New York Times*, April 13, 1930.

p. 35   **He planned to live to be 100**   "Ford Adopts Diet to Extend His Life," *New York Times*, March 5, 1930.

p. 36   **The school was a pastoral vision**   Eunice Fuller Barnard, "Henry Ford Invents a School," *New York Times*, April 13, 1930.

p. 36   **a doctrine that the processes of life are not explicable by the laws of physics and chemistry alone and that life is in some part self-determining**   http://www.merriam-webster.com/dictionary/vitalism.

Chapter 3

p. 39   **Irma S. Rombauer's self-published 1931 cookbook**   Irma S. Rombauer, *The Joy of Cooking: A Facsimile of the First Edition 1931* (New York: Scribner, 1998), 1.

p. 40   **US food administrator Herbert Hoover testified before a subcommittee**   George Asbury Stephens, *Report of the Federal Trade Commission on Sugar Supply and Prices* (Washington: Government Printing Office, 1920), 62.

p. 40   ***Harper's Weekly* had labeled it our "national drink,"**   Mary Gay Humphreys, "The Evolution of the Soda Fountain," *Harper's Weekly*, November 21, 1891.

p. 40   **As Tom Standage describes**   Tom Standage, *A History of the World in 6 Glasses* (New York: Walker, 2005).

p. 42   **new and extremely popular "all you can eat" restaurants**   Eunice Fuller Barnard, "'All You Can Eat'—And What Is Chosen," *New York Times*, February 28, 1932.

p. 42   **devise elaborate patisseries**   Ibid.

p. 42   **Eunice Fuller Barnard suggested**   Eunice Fuller Barnard, "New Styles in Diet as Well as Dress," *New York Times*, November 1, 1931.

p. 42   **American farmers were drowning in surplus wheat**   "Wheat in 'the Seventies,'" *New York Times*, September 17, 1930.

p. 42   **much of the blame was placed on women and their desire to "reduce."**   "Blames Dieting Fad for Wheat Surplus," *New York Times*, May 17, 1931; and "Women Expected to Eat into Wheat Surplus to Restore Curves for Eugenie Silhouette," *New York Times*, September 26, 1931.

p. 42   **organize a counterpropaganda**   "Blames Dieting Fad for Wheat Surplus."

p. 42   **Carl Malmberg thought it ironic**   Carl Malmberg, *Diet and Die* (New York: Hillman-Curl, 1935), 8.

p. 43   **Ruth Atwater**   Harvey Levenstein, *Paradox of Plenty* (Berkeley, CA: University of California Press, 2003), 15.

p. 43   **rich in Dextrose**   Corn Products Refining Company, "Karo syrup," in *All-American Ads of the '30s*, ed. Jim Heimann (Cologne, Germany: Taschen, 2003), 511.

p. 43   **Baby Ruth candy bars were advertised**   Ibid., 537.

p. 44   ***Larousse Gastronomique***   Prosper Montagné, *Larousse Gastronomique* (New York: Crown, 1961).

p. 44   **Eunice Fuller Barnard wrote**   Eunice Fuller Barnard, "In Food, Also, a New Fashion Is Here," *New York Times*, May 4, 1930.

p. 45   **a typical budget of $8 a week to feed a family of four**   Print advertisements emphasized limited food budgets. An October 1935 ad for Royal Baking Powder that ran in *Parents'* magazine featured a housewife saying that with only $8 a week to feed four people, she couldn't afford baking failures. An April 1935 ad for the same product in the same publication quotes a bride spending 35 cents a day on food as saying that she needed a guarantee that the chocolate cake her husband loves will be perfect.

pp. 45–46   **Carl Malmberg published an exposé of these senseless fad diets**   Malmberg, *Diet and Die*, 21.

p. 46   **no single subject**   Malmberg, *Diet and Die*, 8.

p. 46   **the Henry Ford–endorsed Hay Diet**   Malmberg, *Diet and Die*, 66.

p. 46   **Logan Clendening, MD, condemned the diet**   Logan Clendening, "Today's Health Talk," *Washington Post*, April 19, 1937.

p. 46   **haywire**   Ida Jean Kain, "Your Figure, Madame!" *Atlanta Constitution*, October 19, 1937.

p. 46   **Malmberg predicted the Atkins low-carb versus Pritikin low-fat wars**   Malmberg, *Diet and Die*, 66.

p. 46   **A plan involving bananas and skim milk**   "Bananas Boom with Popularity of a New Diet," *Washington Post*, May 16, 1934; and "Skim Milk, Banana Diet Cuts Weight," *Washington Post*, June 1, 1934.

p. 47   **Paul Whiteman**   Antoinette Donnelly, "Whiteman Drops His Burden and Tells the World How He Did It," *Chicago Daily Tribune*, August 23, 1933.

p. 47   **Eventually even Ida Jean Kain joined the party.**   Ida Jean Kain, "Your Figure, Madame! Reducing Made Easy By Starting Meal with Half a Head of Lettuce, Thoroughly Chewed," *Washington Post*, April 20, 1938.

Chapter 4

p. 49   **the most effective means of weight loss ever developed**   W. A. Evans, "How to Keep Well," *Chicago Daily Tribune*, April 16, 1934.

p. 49   **Brady was no longer so sure about the drug**   William Brady, "Personal Health Service: The New Reduction Medicine Kills a Person Here and There," *Los Angeles Times*, June 21, 1934.

p. 49   **Emory University scientists**   "Science Finds Cause of Strange Malady," *Atlanta Constitution*, June 21, 1934.

p. 49   **W. G. Campbell, head of the FDA**   "Reducing Aids Held Perilous," *Washington Post*, July 20, 1934.

p. 49   **Some underwent surgery**   "War on Fat Cures Open," *Los Angeles Times*, January 23, 1936.

p. 49   **Two Cleveland physicians**   Ibid.

p. 49   **congenital deformities**   "Deformities Laid to Reducing Drug," *New York Times*, June 7, 1936.

p. 49   **In 1938, a new law was passed**   "Invokes Advertising Law," *New York Times*, September 9, 1938.

p. 50   **pills that were handed out**   German troops were given a similar drug called Pervitin that is still available today and the cause of a current "drug problem" in the Czech Republic.

p. 50   **8 percent of *all* prescriptions were being written for amphetamines**   Jonathan Spivak, "FDA Will Seek Strict Limits on 'Pep Pills,' Curbing Use for Obesity, Nervous Problems," *Wall Street Journal*, May 14, 1970.

p. 50   **Marmola may cause a user to drop dead**   "Medicine: Marmola Silenced," *Time*, June 3, 1935.

p. 50   **Dr. Stoll's Diet Aid**   Carl Malmberg, *Diet and Die* (New York: Hillman-Curl, 1935), 135.

Chapter 5

p. 52   **the sentiment was no longer hyperbole**   H. J. Nelson, "The Trader," *Barron's*, January 1, 1940; "Auto Industry in 1940 Said to Have One of the Best Years in Its History," *Wall Street Journal*, January 2, 1940; "Retailers Predict 7-10% Rise for 1941," *New York Times*, December 29, 1940; and "Retail Trading Reflects Strong Consumer Demand," *Atlanta Constitution*, February 25, 1940.

p. 53   **required 200,000 tons of US food a month**   "Billion Asked for 5-Month Food Supply for England," *Washington Post*, September 24, 1941; and "Foreign News: Empty Cupboards," *Time*, June 2, 1941.

p. 53   **victory gardens**   Harvey Levenstein, *Paradox of Plenty* (Berkeley, CA: University of California Press, 2003), 85; and "Victory Gardens to Bloom in U.S.," *New York Times*, January 12, 1942.

p. 53   **a return to canning**   Levenstein, *Paradox of Plenty*, 85.

p. 53   **old-fashioned housekeeping methods for the housewife of today**   "Women Are Urged to Conserve Food," *New York Times*, November 7, 1941.

p. 53   **The hoarding of clothing and food began almost immediately after the declaration**

of war Ida Jean Kain, "Food Hoarding Unnecessary and Unwise," *Washington Post*, December 29, 1941; and W. J. Enright, "Hoarding Reduces Supplies of Goods," *New York Times*, February 22, 1942.

p. 54 **during the sugar surplus summer of 1941, it had been considered unpatriotic to take less than 3 teaspoons in your coffee** Charles E. Egan, "Nation Used to Abundance 'Kicks' Little at Rationing," *New York Times*, February 28, 1943. One teaspoon had been to help diminish the American surplus. The other two had been for Cuba and the Philippines, which before the war had also had sugar to spare. However, during the war Cuba's sugar was converted into alcohol for use in manufacturing explosives and the Philippines were cut off from trade.

p. 54 **There was no longer an easy willingness to "tighten the belt"** Levenstein, *Paradox of Plenty*, 80.

p. 54 **a family of four could have 8 pounds of sugar in the cupboard at any given time** "Register Today for Sugar!" *Chicago Daily Tribune*, May 4, 1942.

p. 54 **restrictions would probably improve the American diet** Clive M. McCay, "America Is Learning What to Eat," *New York Times*, March 28, 1943.

p. 55 **80 percent of American housewives didn't know the difference between a vitamin and a calorie** Hillel Schwartz, *Never Satisfied: A Cultural History of Diets, Fantasies, and Fat* (New York: Free Press, 1986), 228–9.

p. 55 **Benjamin Gayelord Hauser** Carl Malmberg, *Diet and Die* (New York: Hillman-Curl, 1935), 77–82; Benjamin Gayelord Hauser, *Look Younger, Live Longer* (New York: Farrar, Straus, 1951); and Adelaide Young, "Magic Beans," *Washington Post*, December 13, 1942.

p. 56 **limiting Americans' food intake could only improve their waistlines** Young, "Magic Beans."

p. 56 **Rationing was in effect wherever food was served** John Maccormac, "16 Points a Week," *New York Times*, March 25, 1943; Christine Sadler, "Butter 8 Points; Also Most Popular Pre-Ration Cuts of Steaks, Chops," *Washington Post*, March 25, 1943; and "Meat Ration Held in Ample Protein," *New York Times*, March 25, 1943.

p. 57 **By 1943, rationing and food shortages resulted in a strong black market** "Food Black Market Is Imminent in City," *New York Times*, February 28, 1943; "Mayor LaGuardia Assails Wartime Foodleggers," *Washington Post*, March 1, 1943; "Empty Cupboards," *Time*, June 2, 1941; "Meat for Holidays Is Scarce," *New York Times*, April 15, 1946; and Levenstein, *Paradox of Plenty*, 99.

p. 57 **foodleggers slaughtered animals in Canada and smuggled the meat across the border** "Canadian Meat Smuggled Over Border to U.S.," *Chicago Daily Tribune*, April 17, 1946.

p. 58 **much of Europe was suffering from serious food shortages** Marquis Childs, "Food for Europe," *New York Times*, April 24, 1945.

p. 58 **A series of articles written by nutritionist Ida Jean Kain** Ida Jean Kain, "Lady, Can You Spare 10 Pounds?" *Washington Post*, January 30, 1946.

Chapter 6

p. 60 **Fannie Hurst** Fannie Hurst, *No Food with My Meals* (New York: Harper and Brothers, 1935); and Fannie Hurst, *Anatomy of Me: A Wonderer in Search of Herself* (Garden City, NY: Doubleday, 1958).

p. 61 **their marriage was kept secret** "Novelist Reveals Her 5-Year Trial Marriage," *Chicago Daily Tribune*, May 4, 1920; and "Fannie Hurst Wed; Hid Secret 5 Years," *New York Times*, May 4, 1920.

p. 61 **We believe in love but not Free Love** Ibid.

p. 62 **We had it nice** "Fannie Hurst, Popular Author of Romantic Stories, Dies at 78," *New York Times*, February 24, 1968.

p. 62 **when Peary left New York City by ship in his quest to reach the North Pole** Jim Rasenberger, *America, 1908* (New York: Scribner, 2007), 152–153.

p. 63 **it was not unusual for human "living specimens" to be shipped halfway across the world** Gísli Pálsson, *Travelling Passions: The Hidden Life of Vilhjalmur Stefansson*, ed. Keneva Kunz (Hanover, NH: Dartmouth College Press, 2005), 177.

p. 63   **He gave up on exploring**   "Stefansson Quits Exploring, Leaving Field to Airmen," *New York Times*, January 20, 1924.

p. 63   **the last of the dog team explorers**   "Vilhjalmur Stefansson, 82, Dies; Led Many Expeditions in Arctic," *New York Times*, August 27, 1962.

p. 63   **he was her lover for more than 17 years**   Pálsson, *Travelling Passions*, 189.

p. 63   **in a series of articles for *Harper's Monthly***   Vilhjalmur Stefansson, "Adventures in Diet: Part I," *Harper's Monthly*, November 1935.

p. 64   **Stefansson, who said he lived on only fish or meat for an aggregate of more than 5 years**   Ibid.; Vilhjalmur Stefansson, *Not by Bread Alone* (New York: Macmillan, 1946), 52; and Walter S. McClellan and Eugene F. Du Bois, "Clinical Calorimetry. XLV. Prolonged Meat Diets with a Study of Kidney Function and Ketosis," *Journal of Biological Chemistry* 87 (1930): 651–68; http://www.jbc.org/cgi/reprint/87/3/651.pdf. McClellan and Du Bois report that Stefansson lived exclusively on meat for 9 years, on and off.

p. 64   **he mentions the vegetarian diet famously followed by George Bernard Shaw as an example**   Stefansson, *Not by Bread Alone*, 11.

p. 64   **Americans were consuming 40 to 60 fewer pounds of meat annually in the 1930s than in the 1830s**   Gary Taubes, *Good Calories, Bad Calories: Fats, Carbs, and the Controversial Science of Diet and Health* (New York: Anchor Books, 2008), 11.

p. 65   **The IAMP, which had a physician on the committee as well, was given warning**   Vilhjalmur Stefansson, "Adventures in Diet: Part II," *Harper's Monthly*, December 1935.

p. 65   **any loss of weight was due to diminished food intake**   McClellan and Du Bois, "Clinical Calorimetry. XLV."

p. 66   **Stefansson had once felt ill until his craving for calf's brain was satisfied**   Ibid.

p. 66   **They consumed foods rich in vitamins and minerals**   A recipe booklet published circa 1950 to market organ meats for the "extraordinary amounts" of nutrients they contained charted the daily recommended dietary allowances (RDAs) and calories supplied by various types. Four ounces of the brains Stefansson craved contained 16 percent of the RDA of thiamin, 8 percent of the riboflavin, 27 percent of the niacin, 14 percent of the vitamin C, 23 percent of the iron, and 5 percent of the calories. Four ounces of liver contained 475 percent of the RDA of vitamin A and 24 percent of the vitamin C; sweetbreads supplied 44 percent of the RDA of vitamin C. *Variety Meats: Recipes for Heart, Liver, Kidney, Sweetbreads, Tongue, Tripe, Brains* (Chicago: National Live Stock and Meat Board, n.d.).

p. 66   **letters from Fannie Hurst**   Pálsson, *Travelling Passions*, 183, 196.

p. 66   **His two-subject experiment is still being used as "scientific proof"**   Vilhjalmur Stefansson, *The Fat of the Land* (New York: Macmillan, 1956), xxvi.

p. 66   **the grandfather of no- and low-carb diets and the muse of Robert Atkins**   Vilhjalmur Stefansson, "Adventures in Diet: Part II," *Harper's Monthly*, December 1935.

p. 67   **now titled *The Fat of the Land***   Stefansson, *The Fat of the Land*, ix–xiv.

p. 67   **more controlled scientific data are needed by all concerned**   Ibid., xiv.

p. 67   **They lost an average of 22 pounds in 100 days**   Taubes, *Good Calories, Bad Calories*, 330.

p. 68   **Pennington had been a disciple of Blake Donaldson, MD, a physician who in the 1920s**   Blake F. Donaldson, *Strong Medicine* (New York: Doubleday, 1962), 35; and Taubes, *Good Calories, Bad Calories*, 329.

p. 68   ***The Friendly Arctic***   Vilhjalmur Stefansson, *The Friendly Arctic* (New York: Macmillan, 1921).

p. 68   **Stefansson agreed that this would do no harm**   Stefansson, *The Fat of the Land*, xxvi.

p. 68   ***Holiday* magazine published a supplement**   Elizabeth Woody, "Eat Well and Lose Weight," *Holiday*, June 1950.

p. 68   **it *should* have been called**   Stefansson, *The Fat of the Land*, xxvi.

Chapter 7

p. 71   **The average life span in 1950 was 67 years**   Gary Taubes, *Good Calories, Bad Calories*, 7.

p. 71   **Americans are getting fat on too much food and too little work**   "Overeating Laid to U.S.; Diet Expert Says We Consume Too Much for Our Easier Life," *New York Times*, April 4, 1950.

p. 71   **Dr. Max Millman wrote**   "Obesity Reasons Given," *New York Times*, August 26, 1950.

p. 71   **Psychiatrist Hilde Bruch, MD, believed**   Hilde Bruch, "Body Image and Self-Awareness," ed. Carole Counihan and Penny Van Esterik, *Food and Culture* (New York: Routledge, 1997), 218–20.

p. 71   **Another hypothesis was that women gained weight to replicate pregnancy, or to avoid it**   Theodore R. Van Dellen, "How to Keep Well," *Chicago Daily Tribune*, March 15, 1951.

p. 71   **Within the decade, psychological profiles of the three most typical types of overeaters would be defined**   Lawrence Galton, "Why We Are Overly Larded," *New York Times Magazine*, January 15, 1961.

p. 72   **A. D. Jonas, MD, stated somewhat similarly**   Alton L. Blakeslee, "Losing Weight on a Full Stomach," *Washington Post*, October 22, 1950.

p. 72   **Edward H. Rynearson, MD, of the Mayo Clinic in Rochester, Minnesota, speaking to a group of insurance-company medical men**   "Overeating Called 'Compulsive'; Diet Held Only Way to Reduce," *New York Times*, October 21, 1950.

p. 72   **the plague of the twentieth century**   Robert G. Whalen, "We Think Ourselves into Fatness," *New York Times Magazine*, December 3, 1950.

p. 73   **it had evolved into a modern way to take off weight**   Hillel Schwartz, *Never Satisfied: A Cultural History of Diets, Fantasies, and Fat* (New York: Free Press, 1986), 205.

p. 73   **a Milwaukee woman named Esther Manz**   TOPS Club, "History of TOPS," n.d., http://www.tops.com/TOPSHistory.aspx.

p. 73   **In those early days**   Jack McMurdy, "They Help Each Other," *Los Angeles Times*, September 6, 1959.

p. 73   **By the end of the decade, there were 30,000 members**   Schwartz, *Never Satisfied*, 207.

p. 74   **Manz wrote a formal letter**   Barbara Cady (president of TOPS), e-mail message to author, April 16, 2009.

p. 74   **members lost more than 430 tons**   TOPS Club, "Fabulous Figures," n.d., http://www.tops.org/SuccessStory.aspx.

p. 74   **In 1951, a *New York Times* reporter enrolled in a typical ad hoc meeting on Manhattan's Lower East Side**   June Owen, "News of Food," *New York Times*, November 12, 1951.

p. 74   **calorie clubs**   "Calorie Clubs Hold First Dance Saturday," *Chicago Daily Tribune*, July 26, 1951.

p. 74   **Group hypnosis**   Roy Gibbons, "Plump Gals Grow Slim in Hypnotic Paradise," *Chicago Daily Tribune*, October 4, 1958.

p. 74   **Hypnotherapist Herbert Mann, MD**   Ibid.

p. 75   **Overweight among American business executives is threatening destruction of the nation's productive capacity**   Roy Gibbons, "Obesity among Executives Threatens U.S., Doctors Told," *Chicago Daily Tribune*, June 14, 1952.

p. 75   **Antoinette Donnelly quickly shifted responsibility to housewives**   Antoinette Donnelly, "Stop Killing Your Husband," *Chicago Daily Tribune*, April 7, 1953.

p. 75   **The Caterpillar Tractor Company in Peoria, Illinois, took swift action**   Gibbons, "Obesity among Executives."

p. 75   **Remarks about "fat folks" were becoming increasingly prejudicial**   "Fat and Unhappy," *Time*, June 23, 1952.

p. 76   **Overeaters Anonymous**   Schwartz, *Never Satisfied*, 210.

p. 76   **Jean Slutsky Nidetch**   Jean Nidetch with Joan Rattner Heilman, *The Story of Weight Watchers* (New York: W/W TwentyFirst, 1970).

p. 77   **The H. J. Heinz Company bought Weight Watchers International in 1978**   N. R. Kleinfield, "The Ever-Fatter Business of Thinness," *New York Times*, September 7, 1986.

p. 78 **Louis I. Dublin, PhD** William Bennett and Joel Gurin, *The Dieter's Dilemma: Eating Less and Weighing More* (New York: Basic Books, 1982), 130–1; and "Louis Dublin, Statistician, Dies," *New York Times*, March 9, 1969.

p. 78 *To Be, or Not to Be* Louis I. Dublin and Bessie Bunzel, *To Be, or Not to Be: A Study of Suicide* (New York: H. Smith and R. Haas, 1933).

p. 78 *The Psychoanalytic Review* **called the work admirable** *To Be or Not to Be—A Study of Suicide*. By Louis I. Dublin. Published by Harrison Smith and Robert Haas. New York, 1933, 443. *The Psychoanalytic Review* 22 (1935): 110–1 (book review).

p. 79 *To make a simple approximation of your frame size* Metropolitan Life Foundation, *Statistical Bulletin*, 64, no. 1 (1983): 5; and William Stockton, "Ideal Weight Is Just an Elbow Away," *New York Times*, July 11, 1988.

p. 80 **Obesity is America's number one health problem** Bennett, *The Dieter's Dilemma*, 133.

p. 80 **He used the Met Life Insurance statistics to link obesity to a shortened life span** Whalen, "We Think Ourselves into Fatness."

p. 80 **as a student, he had done a good deal of research** Bennett, *The Dieter's Dilemma*, 130–1.

p. 80 **Dublin so deeply believed** Bennett, *The Dieter's Dilemma*, 130–8.

p. 81 **Dublin determined this by comparing mortality on policies** Bennett, *The Dieter's Dilemma*, 135.

p. 81 **Excess weight carries very definite penalties in terms of health and longevity** "Liability to Ills Found in Obesity," *New York Times*, October 13, 1951; and Nate Haseltine, "Fat People Die Earlier, Recent Study Finds," *Washington Post*, December 9, 1951.

p. 81 **Met Life stated that the country's high standard of living resulted in the highest obesity rates in the world** "News of Food: Public to Be Half Billion Pounds Lighter If Insurance Company's Drive Is Success," *New York Times*, July 18, 1951.

p. 82 **D. B. Armstrong, MD** Ibid.

p. 82 **The longer the belt line, the shorter the life line** Ibid.

p. 82 **The connection between diabetes, heart disease, and obesity appeared irrefutable** "Expert Reveals Americans Eating Themselves into the Grave," *Atlanta Daily World*, January 30, 1951.

p. 82 **a national health menace** "Pounds of Flesh," *Washington Post*, April 8, 1951.

p. 83 **Kroc opened his first McDonald's** "The Burger That Captured the Country," *Time*, September 17, 1973; J. Anthony Lukas, "As American as a McDonald's Hamburger on the Fourth of July," *New York Times*, July 4, 1971; and William Grimes, "The Way We Live Now," *New York Times*, May 30, 1999.

p. 84 **beef stew luncheons, and Dairy Month** Jane Nickerson, "News of Food," *New York Times*, September 23, 1954.

p. 85 **The feast included powdered orange juice** Harvey Levenstein, *Paradox of Plenty* (Berkeley, CA: University of California Press, 2003), 113.

p. 85 **eggs would be indefinitely "fresh"** Nickerson, "News of Food."

p. 85 **an increase in per capita food consumption of 12 percent over the 1935 to 1939 time period** Bess Furman, "Obesity Is Termed No. 1 Nutrition Ill," *New York Times*, December 9, 1952.

p. 86 **Exercising was said to be useless** Theodore R. Van Dellen, "How to Keep Well," *Washington Post*, December 4, 1957.

p. 86 *Time* **magazine quoted a physician at an AMA meeting in Chicago** "Medicine: Fat and Unhappy," *Time*, June 23, 1952.

p. 86 **Slenderella International reducing salons** Agnes McCarty, "Those Salons of Reducing Offer Expanded Careers," *New York Times*, April 5, 1956; Winzola McLendon, "Got a Weighty Problem? Then Take It Lying Down," *Washington Post*, August 22, 1957; and "U.S. Claims Taxes from Slenderella," *New York Times*, April 21, 1959.

p. 86 **the narrow silhouette of the new and trendy sheath dress** Geraldine Sheehan, "Pleaters Hate It, but the Sheath Delights Milliners and Corsetieres," *New York Times*, November 12, 1956.

p. 86   **Slenderella had competition**   McLendon, "Got a Weighty Problem?"

p. 87   **The RelaxAcizor**   "Fat Marches On," *Washington Post,* February 6, 1956.

Chapter 8

p. 88   **In 1903, he paid $700,000 to purchase the largest piece of unimproved property in New York City available south of Harlem**   "Remarkable Contrasts of East Side Seen in Passing of Ancient Schermerhorn Farm," *New York Times,* July 9, 1911.

p. 89   **Samples of grocery store milk**   "New York's Milk Supply," *New York Times,* January 19, 1902.

p. 89   **transitioned into a graduate university**   "Rockefeller University," *New York Times,* February 12, 1956.

p. 89   **This resulted in two promising new weight-loss strategies**   "New Diets Called Source of Danger," *New York Times,* August 25, 1956; Hillel Schwartz, *Never Satisfied: A Cultural History of Diets, Fantasies, and Fat* (New York: Free Press, 1986), 198; and Roy Andries de Groot, *How I Reduced with the New Rockefeller Diet. Part 1. The Rockefeller Diet. Part 2. The Diet for Gourmets* (New York: Horizon Press, 1956), 23.

p. 90   **Baron Roy Andries de Groot was the Oxford-educated son of a French noblewoman, the husband of the successful British actress Katherine Hynes, and a sophisticated journalist and epicure**   Ibid., xii. "Starve and stuff diet" is a term used by Deems Taylor, composer and member of the famous Algonquin Round Table, in the introduction to this autobiographical diet book.

p. 90   **cut way down on certain foods and gorge on all the others**   Ibid., xii.

p. 91   **eat food. Not too much. Mostly plants**   Michael Pollan, *In Defense of Food: An Eater's Manifesto* (New York: Penguin, 2008), 1.

p. 91   **Americans seem to be befuddled by the enormous variety of processed foods available**   De Groot, 68.

p. 93   **those who need to reduce or think they do**   June Owen, "Food News: Latest Rage for Dieters," *New York Times,* September 20, 1960.

p. 93   **lending the over-the-counter Metrecal the illusion of being an FDA-approved prescription**   "Modern Living: Liquid Lunch," *Time,* October 3, 1960.

p. 93   **Good Samaritan Hospital in Phoenix**   "New Dieting Formula: Four Drinks a Day And No Food at All," *Wall Street Journal,* January 15, 1960.

p. 93   **There had never been a diet craze like this one**   "The Theory of Weightlessness," *Time,* November 21, 1960; Owen, "Latest Rage for Dieters"; and "New Dieting Formula."

p. 94   **liquid meals began appearing**   "Business Bulletin," *Wall Street Journal,* October 6, 1960; and Charlotte Curtis, "Simple Fare Offered Staff of President," *New York Times,* May 20, 1963.

p. 94   **a kind of Spanish gazpacho soup**   "Americana: The Theory of Weightlessness," *Time,* November 21, 1960.

p. 94   **along came Sego**   George Lazarus, "Diet Foods Flavoring Competition," *Washington Post,* September 7, 1965.

p. 94   **a lot of people seemed to enjoy the sensation of chewing**   Dee Wedemeyer, "Metrecal: A Shadow of What It Was," *New York Times,* March 9, 1977.

p. 95   **Tillie Lewis**   Autumn Stamley, *Mothers and Daughters of Invention* (New Brunswick, NJ: Rutgers University Press, 1995).

p. 95   **the 15th annual Newspaper Food Editors Conference**   June Owen, "Experts Predict Rise in Demand on Frozen Food," *New York Times,* October 2, 1957.

p. 96   **Hyman Kirsch**   Benjamin Siegel, "Sweet Nothing—The Triumph of Diet Soda," http://www.americanheritage.com/events/articles/web/20060619-soda-diet-tab-diet-coke-diet-pepsi.shtml; and "News of the Advertising and Marketing Fields," *New York Times,* July 26, 1953.

p. 97   **a Coca-Cola spokesperson said its sales were "almost unbelievable"**   "Business Bulletin," *Wall Street Journal,* August 15, 1963.

p. 97   **the most significant new product introduction in the history of the company**   Philip H. Dougherty, "Advertising," *New York Times,* July 9, 1982.

p. 97   **The problem, according to Marty Solow**   Philip H. Dougherty, "Advertising: The Fat Campaign for No-Cal Drinks, the Saver," *New York Times,* May 12, 1967.

p. 98   **Pommac**   Siegel, "Sweet Nothing."

p. 98   **1-calorie Slenderella**   James J. Nagle, "Packaging Shift Pushed for Cola," *New York Times,* September 22, 1963.

p. 98   **Between 1965 and 2002, our per capita caloric intake from beverages doubled from 200 to 400 per day**   Barry Popkin, *The World Is Fat: The Fads, Trends, Policies, and Products that Are Fattening the Human Race* (New York: Avery, 2009), 57.

p. 98   **Under the name of saccharin**   J. G. Adami, "Saccharin," *American Journal of Pharmacy* 58 (1886): 312.

p. 98   **By 1890, it was being prescribed for both, and used as a preservative too**   Rich Cohen, *Sweet and Low: A Family Story* (New York: Farrar, Straus and Giroux, 2006), 96.

p. 98   **Wiley recalls an unfortunate experience**   Harvey Washington Wiley, *An Autobiography* (Indianapolis: Bobbs-Merrill, 1930), 241.

p. 99   **in 1950, Abbott Laboratories introduced Sucaryl**   "New Sweetener Special Diet Aid," *New York Times,* May 25, 1950.

p. 99   **Neither, for example, could be satisfactorily sprinkled on a weight watcher's morning grapefruit**   In *Sweet and Low,* Rich Cohen speaks of family lore indicating that sweetening grapefruit was his grandfather's reason for inventing Sweet'N Low; see pages 80 and 81.

p. 99   **Eisenstadt immediately switched to his not yet marketed formula**   Cohen, *Sweet and Low,* 129, 134–8.

p. 99   **In 1987, the *New York Times* published a history of sugar substitutes**   "The Bittersweet History of Sugar Substitutes," *New York Times,* March 29, 1987.

p. 99   **only about 15 percent of Americans consume any artificially sweetened products on a regular basis**   Jane Brody, "Artificial Sweeteners," *New York Times,* April 17, 2009. http://topics.nytimes.com/topics/reference/timestopics/subjects/s/sweeteners_artificial/index.html.

Chapter 9

p. 100   **In 1954, the sugar industry hired the Leo Burnett Advertising Agency**   "News of the Advertising and Marketing Fields," *New York Times,* January 12, 1954.

p. 100   **Ted Bates and Company**   "News of the Advertising and Marketing Fields," *New York Times,* February 25, 1953.

p. 100   **Reduce and Stay Reduced**   Norman Jolliffe, *Reduce and Stay Reduced* (New York: Simon and Schuster, 1952).

p. 100   **35 percent of the calories Americans purchased were "empty."**   Jane Nickerson, "News of Food: Health Expert Deplores 'Empty Calories,' Far from Vital Nutrients," *New York Times,* June 16, 1954.

p. 101   **realistic enough to also support the new low-calorie sodas**   Ibid.

p. 101   **Fredrick J. Stare, director of nutrition for Harvard University's School of Public Health, seemingly disagreed**   Jane Nickerson, "News of Food: Chief Nutritional Ailments for Adults Are Obesity and Dental Caries, Says Expert," *New York Times,* May 17, 1951.

p. 101   **General Foods would give Harvard $1 million**   "Food Concern Gives Million to Harvard," *New York Times,* February 14, 1960.

p. 101   **Panic in the Pantry**   Elizabeth M. Whelan and Fredrick J. Stare, *Panic in the Pantry: Food Facts, Fads, and Fallacies* (New York: Atheneum, 1975).

p. 102   **the high priestess of a new nutrition religion**   "Medicine: The High Priestess of Nutrition," *Time,* December 18, 1972.

p. 102   **who could relax with a chilled Manhattan cocktail**   Whelan, *Panic in the Pantry,* 23.

p. 102 **no basis for concern** Ibid., 180–1.

p. 102 **Eat, drink and be *wary*** Ibid., 204.

p. 102 **excessive sugar in the diet was a leading factor in tooth decay** Cynthia Kellogg, "Old-Age Ills Laid to a Faulty Diet," *New York Times,* July 8, 1954.

p. 103 **John Yudkin, MD** "Sugar Gets Role in Heart Disease," *New York Times,* July 3, 1964.

p. 103 **Keys believed there was no conclusive evidence that a diet low in sugar would reduce the frequency of heart attacks** Ancel and Margaret Keys, *How to Eat Well and Stay Well the Mediterranean Way* (Garden City, NY: Doubleday, 1975), 58–59.

p. 103 **no mistaking its role in obesity** Ibid, 57.

p. 103 ***Pure, White and Deadly*** John Yudkin, *Pure, White and Deadly: The Problem of Sugar* (London: Davis-Poynter, 1972).

p. 103 **the public and the scientific community had stopped listening** Gary Taubes, *Good Calories, Bad Calories: Fats, Carbs, and the Controversial Science of Diet and Health* (New York: Anchor Books, 2008), 119–20.

p. 104 **a 1953 Harvard study linked cholesterol to arteriosclerosis** Donald M. Watkin, Eleanor Y. Lawry, George V. Mann, and Max Halperin, "A Study of Serum Beta Lipoprotein and Total Cholesterol Variability and Its Relation to Age and Serum Level in Adult Human Subjects," *Journal of Clinical Investigation* 33 (1954): 874–83, http://www.ncbi.nlm.nih.gov/pmc/articles/PMC438523.

p. 104 **United States had the highest death rate in the world from cardiovascular disease** "Diet Related to Heart Disease," *New York Times,* September 19, 1954.

p. 104 **columnist Ida Jean Kain interviewed Johnson** Ida Jean Kain, "Senator Votes Down Fats," *Washington Post,* September 14, 1955.

p. 105 **White said it was "strongly suspected."** Paul Dudley White, "Heart Ills and Presidency," *New York Times,* October 30, 1955.

p. 105 **Cigarettes were also beginning to be "strongly suspected" of contributing to a high risk of coronary death** Robert K. Plumb, "Cigarettes Linked to Heart Disease," *New York Times,* September 6, 1955.

p. 105 **Jolliffe presented a paper** W. Granger Blair, "Fat Men Warned on Reducing Diet," *New York Times, March* 17, 1955.

p. 106 **his conclusion was startling** "Fats and Heart Disease," *Time,* November 12, 1956.

p. 106 **the disagreement over what caused heart disease and obesity continued** Robert K. Plumb, "Experts Disagree on Diet vs. Heart," *New York Times,* January 16, 1957.

Chapter 10

p. 108 **anticholesterol advocate Ancel Keys was the man on the cover of *Time* magazine** The Fat of the Land. Time Magazine. Cover Story. Ancel Keys, 1/13/1961; Brody, Jane E., Ancel Keys Obituary, *New York Times,* 11/13/2004, www.cdc.org/movies/keys.pdf. "The Life and Work of Ancel Keys; Cohen, Ben. Margaret Keys Obituary, *Minneapolis Star Tribune,* 12/18/2006; Keys, Ancel and Margaret, *Eat Well and Stay Well* (1959), and *How to Eat Well and Stay Well the Mediterranean Way* (1975).

p. 111 **Keys chose to focus only on fat** Gary Taubes, *Good Calories, Bad Calories: Fats, Carbs, and the Controversial Science of Diet and Health* (New York: Anchor Books, 2008), 120.

Chapter 11

p. 113 ***Calories Don't Count*** Herman Taller, *Calories Don't Count* (New York: Simon and Schuster, 1961).

p. 113 **Keys wrote** Ancel and Margaret Keys, *How to Eat Well and Stay Well the Mediterranean Way* (Garden City, NY: Doubleday, 1975), 17.

p. 113 **Vilhjalmur Stefansson also noted** Vilhjalmur Stefansson, *Not by Bread Alone* (New York: Macmillan, 1946), 24.

p. 113   **The absurd recommendation of a 5,000-calorie-a-day diet was likely lifted from Stefansson**   Vilhjalmur Stefansson, *Fat of the Land* (New York: Macmillan, 1956), xxx–xxxi.

p. 114   **Subjects at Texas State College for Women**   Ibid., xxviii.

p. 114   **I would do the right thing to the best of my ability and knowledge**   Taller, *Calories Don't Count*, 10.

p. 115   **The FDA ruled that all of Taller's claims were "false and misleading."**   "Best-Seller on Diet Confiscated by U.S.," *New York Times*, January 24, 1962; and "Dietary Additive and Best-Seller Seized in Brooklyn by the U.S.," *New York Times*, January 25, 1962.

p. 115   **deliberately created and used to promote sales of 'worthless safflower oil capsules**   Marjorie Hunter, "U.S. Official Says Calorie Book Was a Promotion for Capsules," *New York Times*, July 7, 1962.

p. 115   **The plain fact is weight reduction requires the reduction of caloric intake**   Ibid.

p. 115   **Cove sued Simon and Schuster for $6.5 million**   "Simon & Schuster Sues on 'Calories,'" *New York Times*, July 28, 1962.

p. 116   **In March 1964, a federal grand jury in Brooklyn indicted Herman Taller**   James P. McCaffrey, "Fraud Is Charged in Diet Capsules," *New York Times*, March 12, 1964; "Federal Jury Indicts Weight-Control Book's Author, Drug Maker," *Wall Street Journal*, March 12, 1964; and "F.T.C. Examiner Would Drop 'Calories Don't Count' Case," *New York Times*, June 9, 1966.

p. 116   **pudgy Taller**   "People," *Time*, March 20, 1964.

p. 116   **In actuality, he faced a maximum of 50 years in prison**   "Calories Don't Count Author Is Found Guilty on 12 Charges," *Wall Street Journal*, May 11, 1967; and F. David Anderson, "Author of 'Calories Don't Count' Found Guilty of Fraud in Pills," *New York Times*, May 11, 1967.

p. 117   **a popular diet created by the US Air Force**   The diet would be published in a book edited by Evelyn L. Fiore titled *The Low Carbohydrate Diet: The Widely Circulated Diet Usually Called "the Air Force Diet," Now for the First Time with Complete List of Carbohydrate and Calorie Content of All Common Foods* (New York: Nelson, 1965).

p. 117   **Fredrick Stare, who had stated**   Stefansson, *Fat of the Land*, xii.

p. 117   **in a sense equivalent to mass murder**   William Borders, "New Diet Decried by Nutritionists," *New York Times*, July 7, 1965.

p. 118   **Three months earlier**   Dennis Hevisi, "Robert Cameron, High-Flying 'Above' Photographer, 98," *New York Times*, November 22, 2009.

p. 118   ***The Doctor's Quick Weight Loss Diet***   Irwin Maxwell Stillman with Samm Sinclair Baker, *The Doctor's Quick Weight Loss Diet* (Englewood Cliffs, NJ: Prentice-Hall, 1967).

p. 120   **Craig Claiborne was a guest in 1979**   Craig Claiborne, "The Scarsdale Diet Doctor: Scarsdale Doctor Gives Off-Diet Dinner," *New York Times*, March 28, 1979.

p. 120   **Tarnower had been handing out mimeographed copies**   Herman Tarnower and Samm Sinclair Baker, *The Complete Scarsdale Medical Diet Plus Dr. Tarnower's Lifetime Keep-Slim Program* (New York: Rawson, Wade, 1978).

p. 120   **This is a sample of the original meal plan for Thursday**   Diana Trilling, *Mrs. Harris: The Death of the Scarsdale Diet Doctor* (New York: Harcourt Brace Jovanovich, 1981), 37.

p. 122   ***The Dr. DeBetz Champagne Diet***   Wolfgang Saxon, "Samm Sinclair Baker, 87, Author of Dozens of Self-Help Books," *New York Times*, March 23, 1997.

p. 122   **Herman Tarnower had just begun outlining a new book**   Lawrence K. Altman, "Tarnower Was a Busy Physician, Too," *New York Times*, March 12, 1980; and James Feron, "'Scarsdale Diet' Doctor Slain; Headmistress Charged," *New York Times*, March 12, 1980.

Chapter 12

p. 123   **Senate Select Committee on Nutrition and Human Needs**   Jane E. Brody, "Senate Nutrition Panel to Focus on Perils of Being Overweight," *New York Times*, April 13, 1973.

p. 123   **cardiologist Robert C. Atkins, MD, and his book**   Robert C. Atkins, *Dr. Atkins' Diet Revolution: The High Calorie Way to Stay Thin Forever* (New York: D. McKay, 1972).

p. 123   **McGovern and the committee considered Atkins's book**   Brody, "Senate Nutrition Panel."

p. 124   **Senator Charles Percy of Illinois read into the Senate record a statement by Fredrick Stare**   Gary Taubes, *Good Calories, Bad Calories: Fats, Carbs, and the Controversial Science of Diet and Health* (New York: Anchor Books, 2008), 404.

p. 124   **Stare had once written**   Vilhjalmur Stefansson, *The Fat of the Land* (New York: Macmillan, 1956), xii.

p. 124   **If I were a fetus**   Brody, "Senate Nutrition Panel."

p. 124   **sweet sexy science**   Atkins International, Home page, http://www.atkins.com.

p. 125   **common sense observation of every dieter**   "Atkins Issues Reply to A.M.A. Criticism," *New York Times*, March 10, 1973.

p. 127   **The current USDA dietary recommendation is that carbohydrates should make up about 50 percent of your daily calories**   United States Department of Agriculture, "Nutrition and Your Health: Dietary Guidelines for Americans. Part D: Science Base. Section 5: Carbohydrates," n.d., http://www.health.gov/dietaryguidelines/dga2005/report/HTML/D5_Carbs.htm.

Chapter 13

p. 129   **In 1948, he addressed the New York Heart Association**   William L. Laurence, "Rice Diet Held Aid in Heart Disease," *New York Times*, November 17, 1948.

p. 130   **"Needless to say," his son Robert was to write**   Nathan Pritikin, *The Pritikin Permanent Weight-Loss Manual* (New York: Grosset and Dunlap, 1981), 1–2.

p. 130   **In 1974 he cowrote what would be the first of several best-selling books, *Live Longer Now***   Jon N. Leonard, Jack L. Hofer, and Nathan Pritikin, *Live Longer Now* (New York, Grosset and Dunlap, 1974).

p. 131   **In 1980, Pritikin partnered with Ted Barash**   Laurel Leff, "The Selling of Dr. Pritikin's Diet Program," *Wall Street Journal*, December 11, 1980.

p. 132   **the Atkins versus Pritikin debates**   Lynn Darling, "The Fat Feud! Diet Docs Sizzle While Tomes Earn," *Washington Post*, June 11, 1981.

p. 132   **they both made each other look like asses**   Ibid.; and Paul Jacob, "Diet Book Authors Trade Charges," *Los Angeles Times*, October 15, 1979.

p. 133   **He was pronounced dead**   Robert D. McFadden, "Nathan Pritikin, Whose Diet Many Used Against Heart Ills," *New York Times*, February 23, 1985; and Michael Balter, "Pritikin Son Carries On Crusade," *Los Angeles Times*, September 9, 1986.

p. 133   **he had requested that upon his death an autopsy be performed, with the results published in the *New England Journal of Medicine***   J. D. Hubbard, S. I. Inkeles, and R. J. Barnard, "Nathan Pritikin's Heart," *New England Journal of Medicine* 313 (1985): 52.

p. 133   **Senator George McGovern**   Edward Boyer, "Fellow Crusader George McGovern at Rites," *New York Times*, March 1, 1985.

p. 134   **the actual eating pattern of America looked more like this**   Jane Brody, "Monosaturated Fats, Like Olive Oil, Can Help in Lowering Levels of Harmful Cholesterol," *New York Times*, April 25, 1985.

p. 134   **American men, on average, weighed no more than 2 to 5 pounds more than they had in 1927**   Lawrence Galton, "Why We Are Overly Larded," *New York Times*, January 15, 1961.

Chapter 14

p. 136   **Americans were spending 15.7 percent of their disposable income on food**   "Inflation: Changing Farm Policy to Cut Food Prices," *Time*, April 9, 1973.

p. 136   **FATTER FOOD BILLS**   Normal H. Fischer, "Fatter Food Bills," *Wall Street Journal*, January 3, 1973.

p. 137   **housewives organized boycotts and protests**   "Inflation: Changing Farm Policy to Cut Food Prices," *Time*, April 9, 1973.

p. 137　**Lester R. Brown**　Greg Critser, *Fat Land: How Americans Became the Fattest People in the World* (New York: Mariner, 2004), 9.

p. 137　**less expensive imports weren't kept out of the American market**　"U.S. Sugar Quota Reduced as Prices Continue to Fall," *Wall Street Journal*, March 1, 1973.

p. 137　**The *New York Times* published a question-and-answer session**　Philip Shabecoff, "Questions and Answers on Food Prices and Where the Money Goes," *New York Times*, March 24, 1973.

p. 137　**Known as the "set-aside" program**　William R. Doerner, "Time Essay: Time to Plant a New Farm Policy," *Time*, February 26, 1973.

p. 137　**The small farmers argued that they were being victimized**　Ibid.

p. 138　**Earl Butz**　Julius Duscha, "Up, Up, Up . . . Butz Makes Hay Down on the Farm," *New York Times Magazine*, April 24, 1972.

p. 138　**built-in maid service**　Critser, *Fat Land*, 12.

p. 138　**Hawaiian plantation owners were paying laborers a previously unthinkable $3.20 an hour to hand-harvest the stalks**　William Wong, "Sweet 'n' High: Sugar Industry Revels in Record Prices, Some Consumers Switch to Substitutes," *Wall Street Journal*, September 26, 1974.

p. 138　**a 5-pound bag of sugar that had cost 82 cents a year before**　Ibid.

p. 138　**Sugar consumption dropped by only 3 percent**　Jane E. Brody, *Jane Brody's Nutrition Book* (New York: Norton, 1981), 131.

p. 138　**Earl Butz was also forced to resign**　Critser, *Fat Land*, 18.

p. 139　**It is also at least twice as sweet**　George A. Bray, "Fructose: Is It Bad for Our Health?" (commentary, International Life Sciences Institute North America/USDA State-of-the-Science on Dietary Sweeteners Containing Fructose Workshop, Beltsville, Maryland, March 18–19, 2008), http://www.pbrc.edu/pdf/bray-final-paper-080508.pdf.

p. 139　**from fencerow to fencerow**　Critser, *Fat Land*, 10.

p. 139　**It was this overproduction of corn that created the surplus**　Ibid.

p. 139　**food processing company A. E. Staley took the initiative**　"A. E. Staley Mfg. to Boost Corn Processing Capacity," *Wall Street Journal*, September 28, 1973.

p. 139　**Beverage manufacturers like Canada Dry and Royal Crown Cola began tinkering with their recipes**　"Use of Corn Syrup as Sugar Substitute in Soft Drinks Set," *Wall Street Journal*, August 8, 1974.

p. 139　**Soon industrial food processor Amstar committed to a $20 million expansion**　"Amstar to Increase Corn Syrup Output," *New York Times*, August 20, 1974; and "Amstar to Expand Texas Corn-Syrup Unit for Over $20 Million," *Wall Street Journal*, August 20, 1974.

p. 139　**Standard Brands**　"Standard Brands Plans a Corn Syrup Plant," *Wall Street Journal*, October 2, 1974.

p. 139　**American Maize-Products Company**　"American Maize Plans Facility at Decatur," *Wall Street Journal*, November 26, 1974.

pp. 139–140　**More than 1 billion pounds of the sweet syrup were estimated to sell in 1974**　"Commodities: Fructose Has the Sweet Taste of Success," *Wall Street Journal*, May 9, 1984.

p. 140　**profits increased even for small farmers**　Critser, *Fat Land*, 10.

p. 140　**a soda fountain Coke was sweetened with nothing but HFCS**　"Coca-Cola Increases Corn Syrup Content to 100% at Fountains," *Wall Street Journal*, May 9, 1984.

p. 140　**PepsiCo, unable to compete**　Pamela Hollie, "The Sugar Industry's Slide," *New York Times*, December 7, 1984.

p. 140　**By 1990, HFCS had almost entirely replaced all other types of sweeteners in caloric soft drinks manufactured in America**　Bray, "Fructose: Is It Bad For Our Health?"

p. 140　**overproduction drove prices down**　"Staley's Profit Plunges by 49.5%," *New York Times*, January 25, 1982; and "Shot in the Arm for Coke," *Wall Street Journal*, January 4, 1982.

p. 140   **Anyone who uses sugar in his products would be foolish if he were not looking into fructose**   Hollie, "The Sugar Industry's Slide."

p. 140   **the results were in and no one could discern a difference in taste**   "Coke, Pepsi to Use More Corn Syrup," *New York Times*, November 7, 1984.

p. 140   **the consumption of corn syrup increased from 2 to 26 pounds per person**   Jean Mayer and Jeanne Goldberg, "Nutrition," *Washington Post*, October 27, 1982.

p. 140   **a number that would increase to 73½ pounds per person by 2000**   Carolyn Poirot, "Killing Us Sweetly," *Seattle Times*, December 4, 2005. The writer is quoting George Bray.

p. 141   **scientists were just beginning to understand the effects of this tremendous and sudden increase of fructose**   Jean Mayer, "Americans Are Eating Less Sugar; Why Isn't Exactly Clear," *Washington Post*, April 8, 1976.

p. 141   **the US Postal Service stopped mail distribution of diet booklets that advertised fast and automatic weight loss with fructose tablets**   "U.S. Asked to Curtail Fructose Ad Claims," *New York Times*, May 7, 1980.

p. 141   **use had increased to 143 pounds per year**   Bray, "Fructose: Is It Bad For Our Health?"

p. 142   **Between 1980 and 2000, an additional 400 calories per day were added to the American diet**   Ibid.

p. 142   **the brain does not compensate for soft drinks by sending satiety signals that will cause you to eat less of other foods**   Ibid.; and Lenny R. Vartanian, Marlene B. Schwartz, and Kelly D. Brownell, "Effects of Soft Drink Consumption on Nutrition and Health: A Systematic Review and Meta-Analysis," *American Journal of Public Health* 97 (2007): 667–75.

p. 142   **As Greg Critser relates in *Fat Land: How Americans Became the Fattest People in the World***   This book helped me approach, consider, and shape much of the sections on HFCS and palm oil.

p. 142   **palm oil is 45 percent saturated**   Critser, *Fat Land*, 15.

p. 142   **Jean Mayer, a voice of reason once again**   Jean Mayer and Johanna Dwyer, "Trimming the Fat of the Land," *Washington Post*, June 10, 1979.

p. 142   **The popularity of palm oil also frightened the soybean lobby**   George Will, "The Palm Oil Peril," *Washington Post*, March 18, 1976.

p. 143   **Denis Burkitt, MD, suggested that a high-fiber diet might prevent cancer of the colon**   Stuart Auerbach, "Refined Carbohydrates Linked to Increase in Cancer of Colon," *Washington Post*, January 16, 1971.

p. 143   **High fiber became a new diet fad**   Jane Brody, "Personal Health; The High Fiber Diet: What It Can and Can't Do," *New York Times*, March 30, 1977.

p. 143   **Jane Brody of the *New York Times* reported**   Ibid.

p. 144   **Jean Mayer and other health professionals signed a petition**   "Sugars and Cereals," *Washington Post*, September 7, 1974.

p. 144   **In 1980, there were more than 700 over-the-counter brands available**   Brody, *Jane Brody's Nutrition Book*, 147.

Chapter 15

p. 147   **The Metropolitan Life weight charts were adjusted for the first time in 24 years**   "The New Weighing List," *Washington Post*, March 2, 1983.

p. 147   **Ancel Keys agreed with Andres's findings**   A. Keys, "Is There an Ideal Body Weight?" *British Medical Journal* 293 (1986): 1023 (letter).

p. 147   **David Levitsky, PhD, a nutritionist from Cornell University, added**   Philip J. Hilts, "For Healthier, Longer Life Don't Think Too Thin," *Washington Post*, December 27, 1980; Hillel Schwartz, *Never Satisfied: A Cultural History of Diets, Fantasies, and Fat* (New York: Free Press, 1986), 237; and Greg Critser, *Fat Land: How Americans Became the Fattest People in the World* (New York: Mariner, 2004), 97.

p. 148   **smoking had not been taken into account in calculating the new tables**   Jane Brody, "Personal Health," *New York Times*, March 16, 1983.

p. 148   **William Castelli, MD**   "Thinness Linked to a Long Life," *New York Times*, November 18, 1981.

p. 148   **That was the question asked**   "Does Obesity Kill?" *Washington Post*, May 5, 1987.

p. 149   **Four months earlier, the *Journal of the American Medical Association (JAMA)* had published a paper**   JoAnn E. Manson, Meir J. Stampfer, Charles H. Hennekens, and Walter C. Willett, "Body Weight and Longevity: A Reassessment," *Journal of the American Medical Association* 257 (1987): 353–8; and Critser, *Fat Land*, 206.

p. 149   **The following year, *JAMA* published the results of a study**   Don Colburn, "Aging," *Washington Post*, March 15, 1988.

p. 150   **questions about the use of pesticides and additives**   Mimi Sheraton, "Conflicting Nutrition Advice Bewilders U.S. Consumers," *New York Times*, June 11, 1980.

p. 150   **Of the 143 drugs and pesticides the General Accounting Office identified as likely to leave residue in raw poultry and meat**   Sheraton, "Conflicting Nutrition Advice."

p. 150   **The 1980 *Dietary Guidelines for Americans***   US Department of Agriculture and US Department of Health, Education, and Welfare, *Nutrition and Your Health: Dietary Guidelines for Americans*, Home and Garden Bulletin No. 232, 1980, http://www.cnpp.usda. gov/Publications/DietaryGuidelines/1980/DG1980pub.pdf.

Chapter 16

p. 151   **A few of them even contained invaluable information**   For example, a bestseller with credible information was written by *New York Times* journalist Jane Brody. Jane Brody, *Jane Brody's Nutrition Book: A Lifetime Guide to Good Eating for Better Health and Weight Control* (New York: W. W. Norton, 1981).

p. 152   **most ill-advised diet of the decade was Judy Mazel's Beverly Hills Diet**   Judy Mazel with Susan Shultz, *The Beverly Hills Diet* (New York: Macmillan, 1981).

p. 152   **Nothing and everything is fattening**   Ibid., xvii.

p. 153   **the anonymous ABC executive**   Ibid., 225.

p. 153   **Roy de Groot, on the other hand**   Roy Andries de Groot, *How I Reduced with the New Rockefeller Diet: Part 1. The Rockefeller Diet. Part 2. The Diet for Gourmets* (New York: Horizon Press, 1956), 147.

p. 153   **Mazel died not in an automobile accident, but of a stroke**   Dennis Hevesi, "Judy Mazel, Creator of 'Beverly Hills Diet,' Is Dead at 63," *New York Times*, October 27, 2007.

p. 154   **the other best-selling "food combining" diet book of the '80s: *Fit for Life***   Jane Brody, "Warning: The Wrong Nutritionist Can Be Dangerous to Your Health," *New York Times*, April 17, 1988; and James J. Kenney, "*Fit For Life*: Some Notes on the Book and Its Roots," *Nutrition Forum* 3, no. 3 (1986).

p. 155   **Sassafras Herbert**   Sassafras was not the only nonhuman member of the organization—a hamster also joined.

p. 155   **Jean Mayer, president of Tufts University, wrote**   Jean Mayer, "Tough to Swallow," *Wall Street Journal*, October 29, 1985.

p. 155   **When he died in 1994**   John Connolly, "How Bad Was Stuart Berger?" *New York*, April 11, 1994.

p. 156   **about 6% are worth a damn**   Carry Dolan, "I Am What I Ate," *Wall Street Journal*, April 24, 1987.

p. 156   **By the close of the decade**   Cynthia L. Ogden, Cheryl D. Fryar, Margaret D. Carroll, and Katherine M. Flegal, *Mean Body Weight, Height, and Body Mass Index, United States 1960–2002* (Hyattsville, MD: National Center for Health Statistics, 2004), http://www.cdc. gov/nchs/data/ad/ad347.pdf.

p. 157   **hyperpalatable**   David A. Kessler, *The End of Overeating: Taking Control of the Insatiable American Appetite* (Emmaus, PA: Rodale, 2009), 137.

p. 157   **he argues that for the last 100 years, the cultural tolerance for excess weight had "grown especially narrow"**   Hillel Schwartz, *Never Satisfied: A Cultural History of Diets, Fantasies, and Fat* (New York: Collier Macmillan, 1986), 4.

p. 157   **the hostility towards fat extends far beyond physiology**   Ibid., 6.

p. 157   **Ivana Trump, for example, told reporters in 1986**   Molly O'Neill, "The 90's Woman: How Fat Is Fat?" *New York Times*, January 2, 1991.

p. 157   **Fonda**   Schwartz, *Never Satisfied*, 334–5.

pp. 157–158   **the emerging fear of anorexia**   Ibid., 336.

p. 158   **He could not possibly have known**   Jeffrey Levi, Serena Vinter, Liz Richardson, Rebecca St. Laurent, and Laura M. Segal, *F as in Fat: How Obesity Policies Are Failing in America 2009* (Washington, DC: Trust for America's Health, 2009).

p. 158   **By 1985 it was estimated that 25 million people, 90 percent of them female, had tried aerobic dance classes**   Roberta Pollack Seid, *Never Too Thin: Why Women Are at War with Their Bodies* (New York: Prentice Hall, 1989), 236.

p. 158   **credit card debt**   M. J. Stephey, "A Brief History of: Credit Cards," *Time*, April 23, 2009; Seid, *Never Too Thin*, 235–6; and Haiyan Shui and Lawrence M. Ausubel, *Time Inconsistency in the Credit Card Market* [Econometric Society 2004 North American Summer Meetings, no. 176], http://gemini.econ.umd.edu/jrust/sdp/haiyan_paper.pdf.

Chapter 17

p. 160   **The President's Council on Physical Fitness and Sports**   An overview of the volunteer committee's 5-decade history can be found at http://www.fitness.gov/50thanniversary/toolkit-firstfiftyyears.htm.

p. 160   **Shane MacCarthy**   "Shane MacCarthy," *Sports Illustrated*, October 1, 1956, http://sportsillustrated.cnn.com/vault/article/magazine/MAG1131664/index.htm.

p. 160   **MacCarthy was critical of America's young men**   William R. Conklin, "Lack of Physical Fitness in U.S. Blasted by Government Official," *New York Times*, December 14, 1956.

p. 161   **The message of the council was unfocused**   Leonard Buder, "Eisenhower Acts on Youth Fitness," *New York Times*, June 20, 1956.

p. 161   **In 1956, Eisenhower added a citizens' advisory committee**   "Youth Fitness Unit Set," *New York Times*, June 1, 1957.

p. 161   **had neither delivered any blueprint for fitness nor even agreed upon a definition of the word**   Homer Bigart, "Eisenhower Talk on Fitness Asked," *New York Times*, September 11, 1957.

p. 161   **Nixon, who never developed any interest in the project, told MacCarthy**   Ibid.

p. 161   **The Soft American**   John F. Kennedy, "The Soft American," *Sports Illustrated*, December 26, 1960, http://sportsillustrated.cnn.com/vault/article/magazine/MAG1134750/index.htm; and "Kennedy Told to Push Fitness Program," *New York Times*, December 21, 1960.

p. 162   **it was necessary for the council to publish a cautionary warning**   The President's Council on Physical Fitness, press release, February 12, 1963, http://www.jfklibrary.org/Historical+Resources/Archives/Reference+Desk/The+Presidents+Council+On+Physical+Fitness+Press+Release.htm.

p. 163   **In this promising new atmosphere, even Superman was summoned to help**   "Superman Meets Kennedy on Vigor," *New York Times*, August 30, 1963.

p. 164   **What are you doing about your son's nickname?**   "Physical Fitness for Youngsters," *New York Times*, April 10, 1964.

p. 164   **With public school budgets stretched tight**   Anastasia Toufexis, Beth Austin, and Charles Pelton, "Health and Fitness: Getting an F for Flabby," *Time*, January 26, 1987.

p. 164   **the best kept secret in America today**   Ibid.

p. 165   **when an uptick in obesity was reported in France**   Barry Popkin, *The World Is Fat: The Fads, Trends, Policies, and Products That Are Fattening the Human Race* (New York: Avery, 2009), 157.

p. 165   **In 1960, only about 24 percent of adult Americans said that they worked out**   Christopher Redman, Sue Rafferty, and J. D. Reed, "America Shapes Up: One, Two, Ugh, Groan, Splash: Get Lean, Get Taut, Think Gorgeous," *Time*, November 2, 1981.

p. 166   **national obsession**   Ibid.

p. 166   **walking to school decreased by 60 percent**   Claudia Wallis, "Get Moving!" *Time*, May 26, 2005.

p. 166   **American children were exposed to, on average, an astonishing 10,000 food commercials a year**   Philip Elmer-Dewitt, Janice M. Horowitz, Lawrence Mondi, Ken Myers, Bonnie I. Rochman, Martha Smilgis, and Richard Woodbury, "Fat Times: What Health Craze?" *Time*, January 16, 1995.

p. 166   **To counter this**   Ibid.

p. 166   **The national fitness fixation has come off the hinge**   Ibid.

p. 167   **In 1995 America, every age group was heavier than the comparable group had been 10 years earlier**   Ibid.

p. 167   **All of us were stunned**   Ibid.

p. 168   **Oprah said she got her amazing results with Optifast**   "3 Liquid Diet Marketers Told to Alter Ad Claims," *New York Times*, October 17, 1991.

Chapter 18

p. 169   **In 1995, more than 1,300 new fat-free or low-fat products were introduced**   Judith Warner, "Olestra? Quelle Horreur!" *New York Times*, February 3, 1996 (opinion).

p. 169   **Marion Nestle, PhD, in her significant 2002 book *Food Politics*, describes**   Marion Nestle, *Food Politics: How the Food Industry Influences Nutrition and Health* (Berkeley, CA: University of California Press, 2002), 338–57.

p. 170   **Snackwells, to be clear, have no olestra**   Kraft Foods, "Product Detail: Snackwells Cookie Cakes Devil's Food," n.d., http://www.nabiscoworld.com/Brands/ProductInformation. aspx?BrandKey=snackwells&Site=1&Product=4400004754.

p. 170   **In 2003, the FDA said the label warning consumers of olestra's presence in a product no longer was required**   Sherri Day, "Olestra Label Not Required, FDA Says," *New York Times*, August 2, 2003.

p. 170   **Olestra turned out to be a gamble that never paid off for P&G**   Nestle, *Food Politics*, 348–9.

p. 170   **most Americans had wearied of making fat the enemy**   Dan Canedy, "Proctor and Gamble Overestimates Olestra Craving," *New York Times*, July 21, 1999.

p. 171   ***Sugar is toxic!***   H. Leighton Steward, Morrison C. Bethea, Samuel S. Andrews, and Luis A. Balart, *Sugar Busters!* (New York: Ballantine, 1998), 3.

p. 171   **a noble effort by Myrna Melling**   Dean Ornish, *Eat More, Weigh Less* (New York: HarperCollins, 1993), 343.

Chapter 19

p. 172   ***The Redux Revolution***   Sheldon Levine, *The Redux Revolution* (New York: William Morrow, 1996).

p. 172   **In September, *Time* put the drug on its cover**   Michael D. Lemonick, William Dowell, J. Madeleine Nash, Ainissa Ramirez, Brian Reid, and Jeffrey Ressner, "The New Miracle Drug?" *Time*, September 23, 1996. "The hot new diet pill. Redux really seems to work. But is it too good to be true?" is the question asked on the cover, alongside a picture of a woman with a perfect body in a maillot swimsuit.

p. 172   **the fastest launch of any drug in the history of the pharmaceutical industry**   Lemonick, "The New Miracle Drug?"

p. 173   **Eli Lilly, the pharmaceutical giant**   N. R. Kleinfield, "The Ever-Fatter Business of Thinness," *New York Times*, September 7, 1986.

pp. 173–174   **With its patent on fenfluramine soon to expire, Wyeth-Ayerst Laboratories**   Kate Cohen, "Fen-Phen Nation," *Frontline*, November 13, 2003, http://www.pbs.org/wgbh/pages/frontline/shows/prescription/hazard/fenphen.html.

p. 174   **In July 1997, 24 previously healthy women**   Gina Kolata, "Two Popular Diet Pills Linked to Problems with Heart Valves," *New York Times*, July 9, 1997.

p. 174   **Wyeth-Ayerst voluntarily recalled both Redux and fenfluramine**   Nanci Hellmich, "Diet Drugs Pulled Off the Market," *USA Today,* September 16, 1997.

p. 174   **the new millennium began with the FDA being very cautious**   Thomas Gryta, "Obesity Drugs Weighed Down by Past Risks," *New York Times,* March 25, 2009.

p. 175   **the industry's crowning achievement**   Marion Nestle, *Food Politics: How the Food Industry Influences Nutrition and Health* (Berkeley, CA: University of California Press, 2002), 223.

p. 175   **Instead, the FDA had to prove a product *unsafe* if it wanted to recall it**   See Nestle, *Food Politics,* pages 222 to 246 for further explanation of DSHEA and its consequences.

p. 175   **It is currently an ingredient in a variety of weight-loss products, including Apidexin**   See the Apidexin Web site at http://www.apidexin.com.

p. 175   **One of the most widely consumed of these products was Metabolife 356**   Mary Duffy, "Side Effects Raise Flag on Dangers of Ephedra," *New York Times,* October 12, 1999; and "An Indelible Stain: Metabolife Founder Can't Erase the Past," *San Diego Union-Tribune,* October 9, 1999.

p. 176   **He responded that Metabolife 356 was "claims free."**   Onell R. Soto, "Metabolife Co-Owner Admits Charges," *San Diego Union-Tribune,* October 2, 2005.

p. 176   **As early as 1993, physicians began to submit hundreds of negative reports to the FDA**   Nestle, *Food Politics,* 283.

p. 176   **In 2003, Stephen Bechler**   Douglas Kalman, "Ephedra Is Risky, but So Is Lack of Testing for Stressed Players," *New York Times,* March 16, 2003; and T. J. Quinn, "Ephedra Ban 'Not Enough': Bechlers, Docs Rip 1994 Law," *New York Daily News,* December 31, 2003.

p. 176   **ephedra was linked to 10 deaths, 13 cases of permanent disability, and more than 60 other serious adverse effects**   Jane Brody, "Weight Loss Drugs: Hoopla and Hype," *New York Times,* April 24, 2007.

p. 176   **Ellis, as it turned out, had lied to the FDA**   Soto, "Metabolife Co-Owner Admits Charges."

p. 176   **In 2008, Ellis pleaded guilty**   Mike Freeman, "Metabolife's former CEO sentenced to 6 months," *San Diego Union-Tribune,* June 10, 2008.

p. 177   **Hydroxycut**   US Food and Drug Administration, "Questions and Answers: Hydroxycut," September 14, 2009, http://www.fda.gov/NewsEvents/PublicHealthFocus/ucm155837.htm; and Natasha Singer, "Hydroxycut Diet Aids Recalled After Warning," *New York Times,* May 1, 2009.

p. 177   **asked whether the FDA had "adequate authority**   Singer, "Hydroxycut Diet Aids Recalled After Warning."

p. 178   **The difference between a drug and a supplement**   www.fda.gov/Food/LabelingNutrition/LabelClaims/ucm111447.htm, www.fda.gov/Food/DietarySupplements/ConsumerInformation/ucm110417.htm; and Nestle, *Food Politics,* 229.

p. 178   **in 2006, Americans spent $1.3 billion dollars**   Brody, "Weight Loss Drugs: Hoopla and Hype."

Chapter 20

p. 179   **recommended only for obese men and women with body mass indexes (BMIs) of greater than 35**   Barry Popkin, *The World Is Fat: The Fads, Trends, Policies, and Products That Are Fattening the Human Race* (New York: Avery, 2009), 116–7.

p. 180   **analysis of almost 14,000 postoperative patients concluded that mortality is rare**   Mario Morino, Mauro Toppino, Pietro Forestieri, Luigi Angrisani, Marco Ettore Allaix, and Nicola Scopinaro, "Mortality After Bariatric Surgery: Analysis of 13,871 Morbidly Obese Patients from a National Registry," *Annals of Surgery* 246 (2007): 1002–9.

p. 180   **another large study placed it at 0.25 percent**   Lars Sjöström, Anna-Karin Lindroos, Markku Peltonen, Jarl Torgerson, Claude Bouchard, Björn Carlsson, Sven Dahlgren, Bo Larsson, Kristina Narbro, Carl David Sjöström, Marianne Sullivan, and Hans Wedel, "Lifestyle, Diabetes, and Cardiovascular Risk Factors 10 Years after Bariatric Surgery," *New England Journal of Medicine* 351 (2004): 2683–93.

p. 180 **World Health Organization (WHO) stated** Claudia Bambs, Jaime Cerda, and Alex Escalona, "Morbid Obesity in a Developing Country: The Chilean Experience," *Bulletin of the World Health Organization* 86 (2008): 813–4, http://www.who.int/bulletin/volumes/86/10/07-048785.pdf.

p. 180 **largest study to date** Sjöström, "Lifestyle, Diabetes, and Cardiovascular Risk Factors 10 Years after Bariatric Surgery."

p. 180 **In 2008, CBS's *60 Minutes* aired a piece on the procedure** CBS, "The Bypass Effect on Diabetes, Cancer," *60 Minutes*, April 20, 2008, http://www.cbsnews.com/stories/2008/04/17/60minutes/main4023451.shtml.

p. 181 **insurance companies often cover the cost** Stephen J. Dubner and Steven D. Levitt, "The Stomach-Surgery Conundrum," *New York Times*, November 18, 2007; and Popkin, *The World Is Fat*, 118.

p. 181 **negative results have been reported** Francis Delpeuch, Bernard Maire, Emmanuel Monnier, and Michelle Holdsworth, *Globesity: A Planet Out of Control?* (Sterling, VA: Earthscan, 2009), 106; and Mayo Clinic Staff, "Gastric Bypass Surgery," October 2, 2009, http://www.mayoclinic.com/health/gastric-bypass/MY00825.

p. 181 **success rate for these surgeries is less than 100 percent** CBS, "The Bypass Effect on Diabetes, Cancer."

p. 181 **WHO reports an 89 percent reduction in the risk of premature death** Bambs, "Morbid Obesity in a Developing Country."

p. 182 **According to the Centers for Disease Control and Prevention, 58 percent of obese patients are never offered any advice about weight loss** Delpeuch, *Globesity*, 108.

p. 182 **It is an interesting argument** See Bruce Ross, "Fat or Fiction," in *The Obesity Epidemic: Science, Morality and Ideology*, ed. Michael Gard and Jan Wright (New York: Taylor and Francis, 2005), 94–5. Ross argues that calling obesity a disease would be similar to calling short stature a disease because there is a correlation between short stature and heart disease in men.

p. 182 **obesity is "probably not" the result of a metabolic defect** Frank Hu, "Metabolic and Hormonal Predictors of Obesity," in *Obesity Epidemiology*, ed. Frank B. Hu (New York: Oxford University Press, 2008), 393.

p. 182 **adults do have brown fat cells** Aaron M. Cypess, Sanaz Lehman, Gethin Williams, Ilan Tal, Dean Rodman, Allison B. Goldfine, Frank C. Kuo, Edwin L. Palmer, Yu-Hua Tseng, Alessandro Doria, Gerald M. Kolodny, and C. Ronald Kahn, "Identification and Importance of Brown Adipose Tissues in Adult Humans," *New England Journal of Medicine* 360 (2009): 1509–17.

p. 183 **It seemed plausible that if humans were injected with leptin** Delpeuch, *Globesity*, 103.

p. 184 **The FDA has been tracking safety issues related to these products** US Food and Drug Administration, "FDA Issues Early Communication about Ongoing Safety Review of Weight Loss Drug Orlistat: Review Includes Both Prescription Drug Xenical and OTC Drug Alli," August 24, 2009, http://www.fda.gov/NewsEvents/Newsroom/PressAnnouncements/ucm180057.htm (news release).

p. 184 **There is a lot of controversy surrounding the drug** Delpeuch, *Globesity*, 105.

p. 184 **The conclusion about the currently available drugs** Ibid., 104. The authors' conclusions reflect those reported in an in-depth review: Diana Rucker, Raj Padwal, Stephanie K. Li, Cintia Curioni, and David C. W. Lau, "Long Term Pharmacotherapy for Obesity and Overweight: Updated Meta-Anaylsis," *British Medical Journal* 335 (2007): 1194–9.

p. 185 **The FDA denied it US approval in 2007 after five people in a trial of 36,000 committed suicide** Eric Hagerman, "Hunting the Elusive Fat Pill," *Popular Science*, March 2009, http://www.popsci.com/scitech/article/2009-02/hunting-elusive-fat-pill.

p. 185 **A small trial showed an average weight loss** NeuroSearch, Tesofensine, n.d., http://www.neurosearch.dk/Default.aspx?ID=118.

p. 185 **a larger trial is under way** Hagerman, "Hunting the Elusive Fat Pill."

Chapter 21

p. 187 **the use of antidepressants doubled** Bloomberg News, "U.S. Antidepressant Use Increases, Study Finds," *New York Times*, August 3, 2009.

p. 187 **Susan Allport, author of *The Queen of Fats*** Susan Allport, *The Queen of Fats: Why Omega-3s Were Removed from the Western Diet and What We Can Do to Replace Them* (Berkeley, CA: University of California Press, 2006).

p. 188 **annual report that analyzes obesity trends in the United States** Rebecca St. Laurent and Laura M. Segal, *F as in Fat: How Obesity Policies Are Failing in America 2009* (Washington, DC: Trust for America's Health, 2009), http://healthyamericans.org/reports/obesity2009/Obesity2009Report.pdf.

p. 189 **best-selling 2009 book, *The End of Overeating*** David A. Kessler, *The End of Overeating: Taking Control of the Insatiable American Appetite* (Emmaus, PA: Rodale, 2009).

p. 190 **Hardee's Monster Thickburgers** Ibid., 86.

Chapter 22

p. 191 **neuroscientist Paul Ernsberger, PhD; attorney Paul Campos; and physiologist Glenn Gaesser, PhD** Paul Campos, Abigail Saguy, Paul Ernsberger, Eric Oliver, and Glenn Gaesser, "The Epidemiology of Overweight and Obesity: Public Health Crisis or Moral Panic?" *International Journal of Epidemiology* 35 (2006): 55–60; Glenn Gaesser, "Obesity, Health, and Metabolic Fitness," http://www.thinkmuscle.com/articles/gaesser/obesity.htm; and Paul F. Campos, *The Obesity Myth* (New York: Gotham Books, 2004).

p. 191 **a tremendous body of research linking obesity to life-threatening diseases and shortened life spans** For an extensive bibliography, as well as an elegant rebuttal of the "obesity myth," see Soowon Kim and Barry M. Popkin, "Commentary: Understanding the Epidemiology of Overweight and Obesity—A Real Global Public Health Concern," *International Journal of Epidemiology* 35 (2006): 60–7.

p. 192 **Some research has even suggested** Roni Caryn Rabin, "Excess Pounds, but Not Too Many, May Lead to Longer Life," *New York Times*, June 25, 2009; Katherine M. Flegal, Barry I. Graubard, David F. Williamson, and Mitchell H. Gail, "Excess Deaths Associated with Underweight, Overweight, and Obesity," *JAMA* 293 (2005): 1861–7; Glenn Gaesser, "Obesity, Health, and Metabolic Fitness"; Eric A. Finkelstein, Derek S. Brown, Lisa A. Wrage, Benjamin T. Allaire, and Thomas J. Hoerger, "Individual and Aggregate Years-of-Life-Lost Associated with Overweight and Obesity," *Obesity*, August 13, 2009 [Epub ahead of print; doi: 10.1038/oby.2009.253].

p. 193 **Two drugs for type 2 diabetes** Eric A. Finkelstein and Laurie Zuckerman, *The Fattening of America* (Hoboken, NJ: Wiley, 2008), 58.

p. 193 **Drugs for bipolar disorder** Duff Wilson, "Weight Gain Associated with Antipsychotic Drugs," *New York Times*, October 27, 2009.

p. 193 **selective serotonin reuptake inhibitors prescribed for depression result in an average 15 to 20 pounds of weight gain** Finkelstein, *The Fattening of America*, 57–58.

p. 194 **60 extra pounds correlates with a 5- to 12-year reduction in life span** Nanci Hellmich, "Extreme Obesity Can Shorten People's Lives by 12 Years," *USA Today*, August 25, 2009.

p. 194 **Health at Every Size** Linda Bacon, *Health at Every Size: The Surprising Truth about Your Weight* (Dallas: Benbella Books, 2008).

Chapter 23

p. 197 **As he approached the entrance, he fell to the ground** Steve Fishman, "The Diet Martyr," *New York*, March 8, 2004.

p. 198 **There was tremendous controversy surrounding his death** Douglas Martin, "Dr. Robert C. Atkins, Author of Controversial but Best-Selling Diet Books, Is Dead at 72," *New York Times*, April 18, 2003; and Fishman, "The Diet Martyr."

p. 198　**New York City's mayor, Michael Bloomberg, made some unfortunate remarks about Atkins's death**　Jennifer Steinhauer, "Dr. Atkins and the Mayor: The Art of Not Saying Sorry," *New York Times*, January 24, 2004; and Winnie Hu, "Bloomberg Offers an Apology to Atkins's Widow," *New York Times*, January 25, 2004.

p. 199　**pretty good for a man who eats that much fat**　Fishman, "The Diet Martyr."

p. 199　**Finally, Veronica Atkins conceded**　Veronica Atkins, "Statements on Atkins' Death," *USA Today*, February 10, 2004; and Fishman, "The Diet Martyr."

p. 199　**the intravenous fluids that he had received had caused his body to swell**　Ibid.

p. 199　**The $1.25 billion low-carb food industry, which had been projected to double in 2004**　Melanie Warner, "Is the Low-Carb Boom Over?" *New York Times*, December 5, 2004.

p. 199　**Martin Luther King had a dream. I, too, have one**　Robert C. Atkins, *Dr. Atkins' Diet Revolution: The High Calorie Way to Stay Thin Forever* (New York: D. McKay, 1972), 294.

p. 199　**"High fat was riding high," Stefansson wrote**　Vilhjalmur Stefansson, *The Fat of the Land* (New York: Macmillan, 1956), xix–xxx.

p. 199　***New York Times Magazine* cover article by science writer Gary Taubes argued**　Gary Taubes, "What If It's All Been a Big Fat Lie?" *New York Times Magazine*, July 7, 2002.

p. 200　**The American Heart Association (AHA) even invited Atkins to be a guest speaker**　Fishman, "The Diet Martyr."

p. 200　**Suddenly, people on Atkins *couldn't* eat all the butter, bacon, pork rinds, and steaks they wanted**　Marian Burros, "Make That Steak a Bit Smaller, Atkins Advises Today's Dieters," *New York Times*, January 18, 2004; and Marian Burros, "The Post-Atkins Low Carb Diet," *New York Times*, January 21, 2004.

p. 200　**Atkins's top employees were in a race**　Maxine Frith, "Fighting for a Slice of the Atkins Pie: The Doctors Who Claim to Be His Successor," *The Independent*, March 22, 2004; and Fishman, "The Diet Martyr."

p. 200　***The Hamptons Diet*** Fred Pescatore, *The Hamptons Diet* (Hoboken, NJ: Wiley, 2004).

Chapter 24

p. 202　**In 1960**　Eric A. Finkelstein and Laurie Zuckerman, *The Fattening of America: How the Economy Makes Us Fat, If It Matters, and What to Do about It* (Hoboken, NJ: Wiley, 2008), 15.

p. 202　**Ironically, when WHO first implemented the BMI scale in the 1980s**　Francis Delpeuch, Bernard Maire, Emmanuel Monnier, and Michelle Holdsworth, *Globesity: A Planet Out of Control?* (Sterling, VA: Earthscan, 2009), 5–6.

p. 203　**In addition to having an increased risk of early death from coronary heart disease**　Finkelstein, *The Fattening of America*, 12.

p. 203　**they would be wasting our time**　Michael Schooff, "Are Low-Fat Diets Better Than Other Weight-Reducing Diets in Achieving Long-Term Weight Loss?" *American Family Physician* 67 (2003): 507–8; Dena M. Bravata, Lisa Sanders, Jane Huang, Harlan M. Krumholz, Ingram Olkin, Christopher D. Gardner, and Dawn M. Bravata, "Efficacy and Safety of Low-Carbohydrate Diets: A Systematic Review," *JAMA* 289 (2003): 1837–50.

p. 204　**Stone Age drawings of the morbidly obese have been discovered**　Frank B. Hu, ed. *Obesity Epidemiology* (New York: Oxford University Press, 2008), 7.

p. 204　**an "obesity gene,"**　Barry Popkin, *The World Is Fat: The Fads, Trends, Policies, and Products That Are Fattening the Human Race* (New York: Avery, 2009), 118–9; and Jeffrey Friedman, "The Real Cause of Obesity," Newsweek Web Exclusive, September 10, 2009, http://www.newsweek.com/id/215115. Jeffrey Friedman, MD, PhD, who is head of the Laboratory of Molecular Genetics at Rockefeller University, has done extensive and groundbreaking research on leptin, a hormone that plays an important role in the regulation of body weight and metabolism. For other studies on this topic, see: http://www.ncbi.nlm.nih.gov/sites/entrez?db=pu.

p. 205   **The Pima Indians**   Finkelstein, *The Fattening of America*, 53–4; and Lorraine H. Marchand, "The Pima Indians: Obesity and Diabetes," May 2002, http://diabetes.niddk.nih.gov/DM/pubs/pima/obesity/obesity.htm.

p. 206   **phthalates**   Jennifer 8. Lee, "Child Obesity Is Linked to Chemicals in Plastics," *New York Times*, April 17, 2009; Sharon Begley, "Born to Be Big: Early Exposure to Common Chemicals May Be Programming Kids to Be Fat," *Newsweek*, September 11, 2009; and Nicholas D. Kristof, "Cancer from the Kitchen?" *New York Times*, December 5, 2009 (opinion). To reduce your exposure to the phthalates that are suspected to be the most toxic, see "How to Avoid Phthalates in 3 Steps," February 4, 2008, http://www.thedailygreen.com/environmental-news/latest/phthalates-47020418.

p. 207   **According to the Children's Environmental Health Center at Mount Sinai**   Mount Sinai Children's Environmental Health Center, "Children and Chemicals," n.d., http://www.mountsinai.org/Patient%20Care/Service%20Areas/Children/Procedures%20and%20Health%20Care%20Services/CEHC%20Home/Overview/Children%20&%20Chemicals.

Chapter 25

p. 209   **Lulu Hunt Peters suggested levying an obesity tax in 1925**   Lulu Hunt Peters, "Shall We Tax the Fat?" *Los Angeles Times*, March 5, 1925. Peters was recommending that those over a certain weight pay higher taxes.

p. 209   ***Smoking and Health: Report of the Advisory Committee to the Surgeon General of the Public Health Service***   US National Library of Medicine, "The 1964 Report on Smoking and Health," n.d., http://profiles.nlm.nih.gov/NN/Views/Exhibit/narrative/smoking.html.

p. 209   **In 1965, when the Centers for Disease Control and Prevention (CDC) began keeping records**   University of Pennsylvania Transdisciplinary Tobacco Use Research Center, "Toll of Tobacco in the United States," n.d., http://www.med.upenn.edu/tturc/pdf/USA_Figures.pdf; Centers for Disease Control and Prevention, "Surveillance for Selected Tobacco-Use Behaviors—United States, 1900–1994," *Morbidity and Mortality Weekly Report Surveillance Summaries*, 43 (1994), November 18, http://www.cdc.gov/mmwr/preview/mmwrhtml/00033881.htm; and Bill Hendrich, "Smoking Rate Is Declining in U.S.," WebMD, November 13, 2008, http://www.webmd.com/smoking-cessation/news/20081113/smoking-rate-is-declining-in-us.

p. 209   **New York has the highest tax, at $2.75 per pack, while Virginia taxes its smokers a mere 30 cents per pack**   Wendy Koch, "Biggest U.S. Tax Hike on Tobacco Takes Effect," *USA Today*, March 31, 2009.

p. 210   **The World Health Organization reports that for every 10 percent increase in the cigarette tax, there is a corresponding 4 percent decrease in consumption**   WHO Report on the Global Tobacco Epidemic, 2009: Implementing Smoke-Free Environments. www.who.int/tobacco/mpower/2009/en/index.html.

p. 210   **increased by only 32 percent between 1983 and 2005**   Eric A. Finkelstein and Laurie Zuckerman, *The Fattening of America* (Hoboken, NJ: Wiley, 2008), 20–1; and Judy Putnam, Jane Allshouse, and Linda Scott Kantor, "U.S. Per Capita Food Supply Trends: More Calories, Refined Carbohydrates, and Fats," *Food Review* 25 (2002): 2–15.

p. 210   **7 percent of those calories come from soft drinks made with caloric sweeteners**   Barry M. Popkin, Lawrence E. Armstrong, George M. Bray, Benjamin Caballero, Balz Frei, and Walter C. Willett, "A new proposed guidance system for beverage consumption in the United States," *American Journal of Clinical Nutrition* 83 (2006): 529–42. Other scientists have estimated soft drink consumption to make up as much as 10 percent of calories.

p. 210   **floozy of the sugar world**   Sally Squires, "Stealth Calories," *Washington Post*, February 6, 2007.

p. 210   **the prices of fresh fruits**   Finkelstein, *The Fattening of America*, 20.

p. 211   **Americans need more exercise, not another tax**   Muhtar Kent, "Coke Didn't Make Americans Fat," *Wall Street Journal*, October 7, 2009.

p. 211   **The Coca-Cola Company has recently formed a partnership**   Jonathan Birchall, "Coca-Cola Promotes Healthier Diets," *Financial Times*, October 7, 2009.

Chapter 26

p. 213   **traveled more than 50,000 miles a year**   R. W. Apple Jr., "A Life in the Culinary Front Lines," *New York Times,* November 30, 2005; Clementine Paddleford, *How America Eats* (New York: Charles Scribner's Sons, 1960); and Kelly Alexander and Cynthia Harris, "Foreword," *Hometown Appetites* (New York: Gotham Books, 2008), xvii.

p. 213   **Crab timbale in New Orleans**   "Century-Old Recipes," *This Week,* July 2, 1950.

p. 213   **Fried turkey**   "Fried Turkey and Fixings," *This Week,* June 18, 1950.

p. 213   **Lobster and Indian pudding**   "Lobster Party," *This Week,* July 16, 1950.

p. 213   **Danish fried pancakes**   "Farm Feast," *This Week,* February 26, 1950.

p. 213   **Blackfish chowder**   "Thomas Tew's Chowder," *This Week,* January 22, 1950.

p. 213   **At a late-November 1950 luncheon table**   Clementine Paddleford, "Vineyard Fiesta," *This Week,* November 26, 1950.

p. 213   **We all have hometown appetites**   Josef Israels II, "Her Passion is Food," *Saturday Evening Post,* April 30, 1949.

p. 214   **One year after beginning her culinary excursions, she wrote**   Clementine Paddleford, "A Year of Good Food," *This Week,* October 16, 1949.

p. 214   **How does America eat?**   Clementine Paddleford, "The Great Food Speed-Up," *New York Times,* February 6, 1949.

p. 215   **81 percent of Americans believed that overweight is a direct result of eating too much and moving too little**   Doug Anderson, "A Widening Market: The Obese Consumer in the U.S.," Nielsenwire, November 2, 2008, http://blog.nielsen.com/nielsenwire/consumer/a-widening-market-the-obese-consumer-in-the-u-s.

p. 215   **A positive development**   Jonathan Banks, "Global Resolution: Eat Right, Exercise More," Nielsenwire, January 6, 2009, http://blog.nielsen.com/nielsenwire/consumer/global-resolution-eat-right-exercise-more.

p. 215   **only 14 percent of those polled rated their diets as "healthy."**   Ibid.

p. 215   **That bit of information was published for the first time in 1727 in London**   Thomas Short, *A Discourse Concerning the Causes and Effects of Corpulency Together with the Method for Its Prevention and Cure* (London: J. Roberts, 1727).

p. 215   **Harvey Wiley, who spent his career**   "Milk Too Cheap, Says Wiley," *Washington Post,* February 12, 1909.

p. 215   **Any man who adds**   "Bar to Pure Food Act," *Washington Post,* December 20, 1909.

p. 216   **Even Harvey Wiley's introduction to Mildred Maddocks Bentley's 1914 *Pure Food Cook Book***   Mildred Maddocks Bentley, *The Pure Food Cook Book* (New York: Hearst's International Library, 1914).

p. 217   **Sales of UPC-coded organic foods increased by 132 percent between 2004 and 2008**   Nielsen, "'Natural' Beats 'Organic' in Food Sales According to Nielsen's Healthy Eating Report," January 21, 2009, http://blog.nielsen.com/nielsenwire/consumer/"natural"-beats-"organic"-in-food-sales-according-to-nielsen's-healthy-eating-report; and Tom Pirovano, "From Obese to Organic—The Next Obsession: Organic, Functional and Local Foods on the Rise," *Consumer Insight,* no. 6, January 2007.

p. 217   **The whiter the bread, the sooner you'll be dead**   Michael Pollan, *Food Rules: An Eater's Manual* (New York: Penguin, 2009), 81.

p. 218   **Delmonico's in New York City closed in 1923**   "Delmonico's," *New York Times,* May 23, 1923.

p. 218   **pledges made by Coca-Cola and Pepsi-Cola to the William J. Clinton Foundation**   Marian Burros and Melanie Warner, "Bottlers Agree to a Ban on Sweet Drinks," *New York Times,* May 4, 2006.

p. 218   **Chain restaurants in New York City**   Kim Severson, "New York Gets Ready to Count Calories," *New York Times,* December 13, 2006.

p. 218   **New York City schools no longer allow bake sales during class hours**   Jennifer Medina, "New Policy Outlaws Bake Sales in Schools," *New York Times,* October 3, 2009.

p. 218   **on January 2, 2010, California became the first state**   William M. Welch, "2010 Laws: From Cooking to Texting: Trans Fats Out in California eateries," *USA Today,* December 31, 2009.

p. 219   **Hopeless Case**   Anonymous, "Hopeless Case," *Washington Post,* March 12, 1909.

Conclusion

p. 220   **A similar triad has been applied to obesity**   Frank B. Hu, ed. *Obesity Epidemiology* (New York: Oxford University Press, 2008), 8–9.

p. 220   **Nicholas Christakis . . . and James Fowler**   Clive Thompson, "Is Happiness Catching?" *New York Times,* September 13, 2009.

pp. 220–221   **The results were published in the July 26, 2007, issue of the *New England Journal of Medicine***   Nicholas A. Christakis and James H. Fowler, "The Spread of Obesity in a Large Social Network Over 32 Years," *New England Journal of Medicine* 357 (2007): 370-9.

p. 221   **Teach Your Children / Feed Them on Your Dreams**   Graham Nash, "Teach Your Children," Crosby, Stills, Nash, and Young, *Déjà Vu* (Atlantic Records, 1970).

p. 222   **Ground beef is not a completely safe product**   Michael Moss, "E. Coli Path Shows Flaws in Beef Inspection," *New York Times,* October 4, 2009.

p. 222   **saved Cargill 30 cents a pound**   Ibid.

p. 222   **its needs were kept within the limits of its resources**   Wendell Berry, "Energy in Agriculture," in *Bringing It to the Table: On Farming and Food* (Berkeley, CA: Counterpoint, 2009), 57.

ACKNOWLEDGMENTS

MY EXTRAORDINARY EDITOR, JULIE WILL, BELIEVED IN THIS PROJECT FROM THE START and unfailingly helped me to conceptualize, shape, and reshape my thoughts to make it so much smarter and better. Julie, working with you has been a wonderful experience. The amazing copy editor Nancy Elgin is beyond thorough—her suggestions and ability to spot glitches are superhuman—and she appears to be infallible. I once told my agent Lynn Franklin that she was "the best agent in the world," because as far as I'm concerned, she is. Ladies—I am so thankful to you all.

Joe Tessitore was so generous with his vast expertise, support, and time that it is impossible to adequately express how grateful I am. I simply don't know what I would have done without him. I am also thankful to Marion Nestle for her encouragement and for taking the time to read and comment on many of the chapters, and to Leslie Garisto for reading the first chapter when the book was in its earliest stages. Leslie, you made so many excellent suggestions and gave so much good advice.

There are so many people at Rodale who were terrific and dedicated to this project: Hope Clarke, Amy King, Christina Gaugler, and Marie Crousillat, as well as technical support from Sara Cox and Chris Coggins. I am happy to be able to thank you all.

Librarians and archivists George Livingston, Douglas Atkins, Marvin Taylor, and Paula Feid gave generously of their time and resources.

The support of family, friends, and colleagues is always invaluable, and never more so than during the solitary process of writing a book. In particular, thank you to Jenny Berg, Bill Bernstein, Diane Garisto, Robert Garisto, Jennifer Greene, Sonya Hamlin, Peter Hubbard, Linda

Klink, Nancy Panzarella, Jon Rodriguez, Meryl Rosofsky, Joy Santlofer, and Gerry Schwartz.

Roger Yager, my wise brother and lifelong advocate, gave encouragement and inspiration, as did my brilliant father-in-law, Bernard Berkowitz.

This book is dedicated to my husband, Bob Berkowitz. He loves to eat, he loves my cooking, he is supportive beyond belief, and he is more than I could have ever hoped for in a guy with whom to share my meals, my thoughts, and my life. I should add that writing a book is much more enjoyable with our cats DJ and Freddie by my side, or at least asleep somewhere in the room.

Lastly, this book is in memory of my mother, Eleanor Yager, who found the time to cook delicious and healthy meals for her family almost every night.

INDEX

Boldface page references indicate photographs. <u>Underscored</u> references indicate charts.

SSRI, 173, 193
Stare, Fredrick J., 101–3, 117, 124, 211
Starvation diets, 118–19, 168, 219
Stauffer System salons, 86–87
Stefansson, Vilhjalmur, 62–67, 113, 124, 128, 187, 199
Stillman, Irwin Maxwell, 118–20, 122, 127
Stunkard, Albert, 167
Sucaryl, 99
Sugar
    Atkins's philosophy of, 127
    calories in, 24
    candy and, 43
    desserts and, 42
    heart disease and, 102–6
    high-fructose corn syrup and, 138–42, 210
    increase in consumption of, 40
    price of, 137–40
    public relations campaign, 100–101
    reducing consumption of, 133, 171
    in soda, 41, 96–98, 140
    substitutes, 96, 98–99, 102
Supplements, weight-loss, 175–78
Sweet'N Low, 96, 99
Synephrine, 177

T

Take Off Pounds Sensibly (TOPS), 73–74
Taller, Herman, 113–16
Tarnower, Herman, 120–22
Tasti-Diet, 95
Tea, 8
Thompson, Vance, 11
Thyroid dysfunction, 175, 182
Tobacco, 210. See also Cigarettes
TOPS, 73–74
Trans fats, 218
Tree lard, 142–43

V

VanItallie, Theodore B., 117, 148
Vegetables, 131, 217
Vitalism, 36
Vitamins, 55, 169
Volstead Act (1919), 40
Vonachen, Harold A., 75

W

Wafex, 85–86
Waithman, Robert, 91–92
Walking, 162–63

Weight
    aging and, 25
    of Americans, 26–27, 85, 134
    charts, 27–28, 78–81
    "comfortable," 29–30
    healthy, 202
    "ideal," 27–28, 79, 119, 147
    longevity and, 24, 26
    measuring, 27–28
    women's movement and, 33–34
Weight gain, 24–25, 189, 193, 203. See also Obesity; Overweight
Weight loss. See also specific diet and fad
    books, 151, 159, 215
    campaigns, 82, 85
    charts, 72, 78–79, 119, 134, 147, 158, 191
    competitions, 30–33
    cookbooks, 107–8
    corporations and, 75–76
    drugs, 48–51, 85–86, 175, 178, 184–85
    fad diets and, 28–29, 34–35, 45–46, 76, 89, 151, 156, 171, 215
    fletcherism and, 12–14
    group therapy and, 72–74, 81–82
    Hurst and, 60–61
    industry, 51, 107–8, 151, 159, 179, 188
    Kain and, 58–59
    leptin and, 183
    mystery of, 36
    supplements, 175–78
Weight Watchers International, 77–78, 188
Wellness concept, 23–24
Wheat, 42–43
Whelen, Elizabeth, 101–2
White, James and Ellen Harmon, 6–8
Whole foods, 6–8, 132
Whole Foods Market, 217
Whole grains, 131
Wiley, Harvey Washington, 14–16, **15**, 82, 98, 215–16
Winfrey, Oprah, 168
World War I diet, 21–22, 72

X

Xenical, 184

Y

Yudkin, John, 103, 127

Z

Zinczenko, David, 215